ACCIDENTS IN THE HOME

Accidents in the Home

Edited by
SANDRA BURMAN and HAZEL GENN

CROOM HELM   LONDON

Published for Centre for Socio-Legal Studies
A Research Unit of the
SOCIAL SCIENCE RESEARCH COUNCIL

© 1977 Social Science Research Council

Croom Helm Ltd
2-10 St John's Road, London SW11

ISBN   0–85664–452–8

Printed in Great Britain
by Redwood Burn Ltd, Trowbridge and Esher

CONTENTS

PREFACE
S. B. Burman and H. G. Genn

The papers in this book were given at a small conference organised by
the Social Science Research Council's Centre for Socio-Legal Studies in
Oxford in June 1976 to discuss the 'Social, Economic, and Legal
Aspects of Accidents in the Home'.* Among other studies, the Centre
is currently engaged in a group of projects which are investigating the
social, economic and legal consequences of serious functional difficulties arising from illness, injury, and handicap. An assumption of the
research is that in order to describe and understand the operation of the
law it is necessary to view legally recognised institutions as an integral
part of the wider social and economic situation of victims and their
families. The work of the Centre on this topic will provide large-scale
empirical data on the consequences of accidents of all types, including
home accidents. It is hoped that this will contribute detailed information
of a type not available at present to policy makers. As part of the preliminary work on this national study, a pilot investigation of home
accident victims was carried out by the Centre in 1974 and the interest
shown in the report of this study by other people working in the field
of domestic accidents encouraged the Centre to sponsor a conference o
on current research in the area.

The papers which follow are contributed by researchers trained in a
number of different disciplines — sociology, psychology, statistics,
economics, law, medicine and social administration — and therefore
bring a wide variety of perspectives to the problems associated with
accidents in the home. All, however, have addressed themselves to a
discussion of current research on this topic in their respective fields, its
findings and defects, as well as the methodological problems associated
with the collection of data on domestic accidents. An introductory pap
paper describes four case histories which illustrate the problems in
practice of investigating the causes of home accidents and the wide
variety of accidents involved. There follows a review of how childhood
accidents are studied by epidemiologists, psychologists and sociologists,
which suggests a need for a change of emphasis in future research. The
third paper discusses methods of studying human behaviour during and

---

* For a list of participants see Appendix.

after domestic fires in order to reduce the risk of accidental death and injury. Existing data on fires in public buildings have also been utilised, and these have interesting parallels for home accidents. The following three papers form a group and discuss the past, present and future work of a section of the Department of Prices and Consumer Protection in collecting national data for improving consumer safety in the home. This work is based on a consultative document on consumer safety, issued in 1976 by the government, and the seventh paper in the book is a critical review of the consultative paper and a discussion of the difficulties in ensuring that research results are reflected in the subsequent formation of policy. The final paper in the book presents some findings of a pilot study of home accident victims conducted by members of the Centre for Socio-Legal Studies. The study investigated how victims cope with the results of their accidents: to what extent support is provided by official and informal sources and by the legal system. Professor E. Maurice Backett, a leading researcher in the field, has provided an overview of the subject in his introduction to the volume. We hope that this collection of papers, which brings together a number of approaches to the study of domestic accidents, will be useful to administrators, policy makers, practitioners and researchers alike.

SANDRA BURMAN
HAZEL GENN

Centre for Socio-Legal Studies
Oxford

NOTES ON CONTRIBUTORS

E. Maurice Backett is Professor of Community Health and Head of Department of Community Health in the Nottingham Medical School. Formerly he was Professor of Social Medicine in Aberdeen. He has done international work on accidents for the World Health Organisation and is the author of papers on epidemiology and the control of accidents.

J. Breaux is Senior Research Fellow with the Fire Research Unit at the University of Surrey. His articles and research interests centre on the modelling and analysis of mass behaviour.

Sandra Burman is a lawyer with the Centre for Socio-Legal Studies and, together with Hazel Genn, was responsible for the Centre's 1974 pilot study on domestic accidents.

Michael Calnan is a sociologist working on the National Child Development Study, and has been at the National Children's Bureau since 1973. He was formerly working on a home accident study with the Medical Research Division of the Health Education Council.

D. Canter heads the Fire Research Unit at the University of Surrey and is Director of the Master's Degree course in Environmental Psychology. He has written various books and articles on the relationships between buildings and the people who inhabit them.

J. W. Dale is Specialist in Community Medicine (Information and Research) in the South East Thames Regional Health Authority. He was formerly Director of the Medical Research Division of the Health Education Council.

Chandra de Fonseka was Professor of Surgery, University of Ceylon, until 1965. Then, as a Senior Research Fellow, he helped to set up the Road Accident Research Unit at Birmingham University. In 1969 he moved to Bristol to establish the Health Education Council's Home Accident Study. He is now working in the Accident Department, Royal United Hospital, Bath.

Hazel Genn is a Research Officer at the Centre for Socio-Legal Studies and worked with Sandra Burman on the Centre's domestic accident pilot study. Trained as a sociologist, she was formerly a Research Assistant at the Institute of Criminology in Cambridge, engaged in a survey of victims of crime.

Bob Page, a statistician, recently joined the Safety Research Section of the Department of Prices and Consumer Protection. He has previously worked in computers and housing research and is currently involved in setting up the national accident surveillance system.

J. L. Roberts is Area Operational Services Administrator in the South Glamorgan Area Health Authority. He was formerly coordinator of the home accident study in the Medical Research Division of the Health Education Council.

J. Sime is a Research Fellow with the Fire Research Unit at the University of Surrey. He has worked on the dynamics of psychiatric settings and is at present investigating the nature of human behaviour in extreme situations.

Michael Wadsworth is a member of the scientific staff of the Medical Research Council's Unit for the Study of Environmental Factors in Mental and Physical Illness, at the London School of Economics, and works on the National Survey of Health and Development as a sociologist. He has formerly worked in the Department of General Practice at Edinburgh University and in the Department of Medicine at Guy's Hospital Medical School.

Caroline Warne is a psychologist currently working on home accidents with the Safety Research Section of the Department of Prices and Consumer Protection; previously she worked on water safety with the Home Office. Whilst working at the National Institute of Industrial Psychology she was largely involved in research related to industrial accidents.

C. Whittington is a Senior Research Officer at the Institute for Consumer Ergonomics, University of Technology, Loughborough. She works as a member of a research group investigating a wide variety of domestic safety problems, primarily from a human factors standpoint.

INTRODUCTION

E. M. Backett

With the continued, though erratic, improvement in the health of our
communities during the last decade or so, a few illnesses and causes of
death have been left to attract our attention and cause continuing
concern. The reason is that they are either not declining fast enough to
keep pace with the general improvement in health, or are remaining
obstinately constant — a few are even increasing. Among the first
group — those not declining fast enough — are accidents, and they
present a particularly complex and exciting challenge because their
understanding and control involves less of medical and more of social
and behavioural insights than do most contemporary health problems;
they are splendidly multidisciplined in nature.

There are, of course, plenty of orthodox *medical* challenges involved
in the control of accidents and the declining lethality of some classical
injuries shows how significant is recent surgical progress. Case fatality
rates are not, however, a satisfactory index of control and their decline,
though a magnificent achievement, is certainly no cause for complacency
for they may conceal the survival of an increasing number of disabled
and handicapped people. Thus, paradoxically, concentration of
resources upon the saving of life after an injury may result in an increase
in cost to society in both human and economic terms and represent a
distortion of priorities in resource allocation. So, while death is still
important and accidental services are vital, we must compute the cost
of accidents using new indices which reflect also the duration and
quality of the life of survivors. If we do this, the use of more resources
in the prevention both of the accident and of the injury may be seen
to be a logical change of emphasis in social policy.

Such considerations have already, of course, forced accident
researchers to concentrate their attention upon prevention, and in this
they are not entirely alone. The House of Commons Select Committee
on Expenditure has recently reviewed the potential of preventive
medicine in general and a recently published Department of Prices
and Consumer Protection consultative document on consumer safety
(Cmnd. 6398) proposes a renewed attack aimed at the reduction of
cost and suffering from accidents in the home. The same objectives
have governed discussions begun in the last two years about our

11

immediate research needs, for example, in the epidemiology of home
accidents (with a view to the development of 'high risk' strategies in
prevention), the accident sequence or process and its sequelae, the
critical features of the safe environment, the growth of 'good' risk-
taking behaviour, the distribution of social and legal responsibilities,
the economic consequences of accidents, and the application of up-to-
date modelling and cost-benefit analysis to the accident problem.
What is now needed is a massive extension of these research ideas and
the translation into policy of such results as are available. The
conference reported in this book records progress to date in the
current attack on home accidents.

One recent development which may assist and speed the process
of resource reallocation and implementation has been a growing pre-
occupation with the place of the consumer in our society. 'Consumerism'
has shown itself in several ways to be important in the control of
accidents. For example, it has become a 'rights' movement in which a
close scrutiny of all standards, guarantees and contracts has been
made with a view to the further protection of the individual and
family in their everyday purchases, servicing, etc. It has emphasised
particularly, the rights of the individual and family to redress and has
reinforced this message through the provision of easy access to legal
advice and by the widespread use of the media to challenge accepted
practices. It has also sponsored the comprehensive and independent
testing of equipment — mostly for use in the home — and has thus
become an important influence in the design of safe appliances.
Finally, and by no means least, from October of 1974 there has been
a new government department — the Department of Prices and Consumer Protection — specifically charged with serving the consumer.
The gathering strength of this movement, as well as the rather belated
recognition of its social and political significance, is not only one of
the prime movers towards the development of new standards of safety
and safety codes, particularly for the home, but may be the stimulus
to more research which is so badly needed. It has also influenced
markedly the growth of the socio-legal studies of accidents.

More subtly, the new consumer awareness, particularly in its wider
context of women's movements and self care, has reflected a growth in
the idea of the responsibility of the individual for his or her health.
Alongside this has come an intense wave of criticism of the irresponsibility of those who destroy the environment, pollute or make dangerous
the countryside or who, for profit or in ignorance, make dangerous
motor cars, houses, clothes, appliances or toys. But in spite of

substantial progress in the last decade, the gap between understanding and actual control of the accident problem is still large. Clearly the renewed attention is not yet enough.

Britain has traditionally taken a very long time to prevent disease — dental caries and diptheria are probably the worst examples, and we are not much better with accidents. The better prevention of some types of accidental injury and death is altogether too slow, for 'causes' are by now well understood and the opportunities for control measures abound. There is perhaps some small excuse for delay in the case of accidents *in the home* where the intrusion of standards and regulations is more difficult and attempts to control behaviour can be little more than exhortations to change long-established patterns. Accidents in the home also present other special features which at once make them a greater and more difficult challenge to society than, for example, industrial or transport accidents, and at the same time may make them more rewarding to study. It is probably in the home that major progress can now be made.

For a very long time home accidents have been considered the Cinderella of research and preventive endeavour. Until the last decade the subject was largely neglected by the doctors (who were, perhaps reasonably, more interested in the care of the injured and anyway were not adept at social engineering) and almost totally neglected by the Research Councils, the economists and the operational research workers. The quality of published material was on the whole poor, speculation (sometimes wildly psychoanalytic) as to 'causes' of home accidents was rife and unsupported by facts, and the whole subject achieved such a low status as to attract little attention and almost no grant support.

The situation has now changed, though we still blunder on in the misuse of denominators; we rarely change the accident situation in detail (even long afterwards), and have done surprisingly and shockingly little to try to understand why some children are 'good' risk-takers while others are very bad (and nothing at all on how to convert the bad into the good). With the change of attitude to home accident research has come a fuller understanding of just how difficult are the problems to be faced. At its crudest, the huge mass of elderly housing, with its archaic heating, cooking and bathing facilities and its lack of light, is enough to deter most research designers. Nor is there anything simple or clear about the behaviour of the people mainly concerned — the two groups who, in behavioural terms, are the most complex in our society: the young and the old — the one learning and the other forgetting.

The home is also the place where most minor sickness occurs to modify behaviour, where chronic illness develops, and where a lot of the alcohol and most of the tranquillisers are consumed.

Home accident research workers are therefore presented with problems of method — the description of (and evolution of hypotheses from) a constantly changing situation in which barely understood behaviour interacts with changing technology. They are presented with problems of criteria — some of the most 'serious' accidents result in almost no injury and may never be heard of. The ones which do result in injury or death are only rarely representative and the circumstances are afterwards so emotionally coloured as to make behavioural analyses difficult. They are presented with problems of access to populations, of sampling, of denominators, of differences in culture, ethnicity, and class behaviour and, finally, with the conjoined and sometimes insuperable problems of confidentiality and legal responsibility. To these problems has recently been added the lively and none too well-directed suspicion of non-accidental injury, which is likely in the future effectively to prevent a true retrospective reconstruction of many accidents to children.

On the credit side, making home accident studies worthwhile is the size of the challenge: the huge cost in human as well as economic terms of home accidents, the relatively untouched nature of the problem (good data are rarely available and might lead to some immediately effective solutions), and the fascination of designing new, multi-disciplined methods with which to approach this classically multifactorial health problem. That early control measures are urgently needed can be seen not only from the lengthening lives of the handicapped, but from the rapid rate of change in building techniques and therefore in standards, the new legal responsibilities of builders and service agencies, the huge proliferation of high speed and high voltage domestic gadgetry, and, above all, from the raised expectations of a population with a critical consumer orientation. This is now a population which is no longer prepared to look upon gas-filled bathrooms, burned children, or falls downstairs as inevitable.

Personal priorities for the study and control of home accidents arise inevitably from a combination of the observer's own interests and skills, from what kind of work is possible and likely to yield useful results as well as, of course, from the seriousness of the problem to be tackled. Because many of today's research teams are government sponsored, their priorities are more likely to be dictated by decisions made in these government departments, often by non-scientists responding to departmental and other pressures and divided by unreal administrative divisions.[1] Somewhere between these two extremes lies a realistic list of priorities for action to deal with this health problem (and many of them are the subject of the chapters which follow). Below are a few examples.

1. *Information systems* capable of providing high quality data (including portable data[2]) for epidemiological studies of all aspects of home accidents, and in particular:
   a) Features of the accident sequence including, for example, descriptions of similar accidents resulting in serious and trivial injury; behaviour before, during and after accidents in relation to the psychological, social, demographic, pathological, physical and other characteristics of the people concerned; detailed clinical and retrospective data, preferably from statutory enquiries.
   b) Characteristics of those at risk, injured and associated with the accident.
   c) Details of the duration of exposure to risk (for the accurate calculation of rates using realistic denominators).
   d) Trend analyses of accidents (secular, regional and other).
   e) Detailed descriptions of the physical environment, including routine reports from engineers on the functioning of apparatus.
   f) Routine access to coroners' reports and the reports of special investigations, including psycho-social investigations.
   g) Application of modelling techniques, variance analyses, etc., to determine the relative contributions of different factors to domestic accidents.
2. *Data about the relationship between accident and injury* and therefore more information about the characteristics of the 'safe environment' for various 'at-risk' groups. The development of standards.
3. *Information as to the characteristics of those who learn to take 'good' risks and those who do not.* The learning of risk-taking behaviour. Family and peer group patterns and whether it is possible to convert from 'bad' to 'good'. The effects of emotional and other disturbance on learned risk-taking behaviour.
4. *The economics of the 'safe environment'.* Costs and benefits of rendering the domestic environment safe. Hazards of a totally safe environment in the learning of good risk-taking behaviour. Predictive models.
5. *The field testing of hypotheses.* Particularly about safer appliances,

check lists, *aides-memoire* and advances in training methods, and
their adequate monitoring.

6. *The application of technology to the prevention of injuries.*
Particularly, for example, the development of cheap, reliable
'sniffers' for toxic gases, guards, switches and 'fail safe' mechanisms.

7. *Rationalisation of research policy.* Particularly attention to priorities
for research and the application of cost-benefit ideas to the allocation
of funds. A special problem is the independence and security of the
government-employed research worker when working in 'sensitive'
areas where blame and redress issues arise. There is a case to be made
for all such research to be conducted through universities or Research
Councils.

8. *Translating advances in knowledge into social policy.* How and
through what institutions is social policy made about health problems such as home accidents? What are the social policy results of
research carried out in government-run units and in universities and
Research Councils? What are the true effects on social policy of
pressure groups, particularly those representing manufacturers?
What actions should be taken at the level of the community
physician in the Health Service who is charged with the control of
home accidents?

It is hoped that these and many similar areas of concern will be the
subject of study during the next few years and that included among all
research protocols will be studies of how best to apply their findings.
Some, but of course not all, of these personal priorities are the subject
of the papers which follow.

E. Maurice Backett

Notes

1. For historical reasons, home accidents due to fires are the responsibility of
the Home Office, while most other home accidents can be investigated by
the Department of Prices and Consumer Protection. Other stupidities are
studies which focus only on injuries to *children* (a thoroughly unecological
approach), those which rigidly and mechanically define the 'home' , which
consider costs and benefits only in economic terms, or which use death as
the main measure of health.

2. E.g. photographic, video, or other recording.

1 FOUR CASE HISTORIES

C. P. de Fonseka

In discussing accidents in the home, it is easy in the welter of statistics to lose sight of the actual people and circumstances involved. In order to make sense of the wealth of data available, it is essential to abstract from case histories the elements under discussion even though this necessary simplification may distort the record of the accident. The case studies described here are designed to put flesh on the statistical bones in the chapters which follow.

In contrast to accidents on the road or even at work, accidents in the home occur in a wider variety of environmental situations and involve a still wider range of articles, people and buildings. A direct cause can sometimes be traced, by detailed on-site studies, far beyond the scene, to a manufacturing technique or a service engineer's misjudgement, and often a multiplicity of causes can be identified. Any realistic discussion of prevention or social remedies must take this complexity of actual accidents into account. The following four case histories of home accidents, two fatal and two non-fatal, have been selected to illustrate these points.

Case History 1: Burns to Face from Gas Cooker Explosion

On the day of the accident the victim's mother cooked the lunch, using the oven of the gas cooker which she had had for about three years. When her daughter aged fifteen years came home from school during the lunch break, she served the meal and turned off the oven. After the meal, which was eaten in a room adjacent to the kitchen and took about half an hour, she lit one gas ring and put a kettle of water on to make some tea. She then asked her daughter to replace in the oven the food that remained from the meal. When the girl opened the oven door there was an explosion which hurled her across the kitchen. She suffered from first and second degree burns to the face with singeing of her hair, eyelashes and eyebrows. When the mother ran in from the adjacent room she saw her daughter on the ground with her hair on fire. The husband was at home at the time and together they managed to extinguish the flames and telephone for an ambulance which took the girl to hospital. She received treatment in the casualty department but was not admitted.

The cooker had been bought on hire purchase from the South Western Gas Board three years earlier, and at the time of the accident the Gas Board was still responsible for its maintenance. The controls of the cooker were in front of the hob at waist height. Each control consisted of a plastic disc with a sleeve which fitted onto a metal spindle. The sleeve and the spindle were surrounded by a steel spring which held the two components together. During the three years that the cooker had been in use, a total of eight control knobs had to be replaced due to breakage. In each instance the breakage occurred to the plastic of the sleeve. As a result of these breakages the fit between the sleeve and the spindle became loose and consequently the housewife lost control of the gas flow to that particular burner. When disgust was expressed at these repeated breakages, the owner was told that his wife used too much force when turning the knobs. The official of the Gas Board mentioned that there were hundreds of cookers with similar knobs giving no trouble at all. A few weeks before the accident in question, the control knob of the oven had similarly failed. It was evident that the plastic had sheared at the edge where it was in contact with the metal spindle.

An immediate replacement could not be obtained but meals still had to be cooked until the Gas Board attended to it. During this period the housewife had to gauge by feel the position of the knob controlling gas to her oven. In her own words, she had to 'keep twiddling the knob back and forth' until she felt the spindle engage and turn. This was the procedure which she had adopted when she turned the oven off after having cooked the meal on the day of the accident. With such a procedure it was quite possible for her to have first extinguished the oven and then inadvertently to have turned the gas on once again. As a result gas could have slowly accumulated within the oven during the time the family were having their meal, and when the girl went to replace food in the oven it is possible that explosive combustion of the gas occurred from the lighted burner under the kettle.

Comments

It was evident from the details of the events that led up to the explosion that no members of the family who participated in those events could be blamed for carelessness. The escape of gas and the consequent explosion could be very clearly attributed to failure of the plastic material used in the manufacture of the control knob. Several possibilities had now to be considered. Examination of the broken plastic showed that it had sheared and crumbled where it had been in contact with the metal spindle. Excessive force, more than the plastic could bear, might in fact have been due to a defect within the mechanism of the tap, making the spindle more difficult to turn. The extra force that would then have been needed to operate the control could have produced excessive shearing forces between the spindle and the plastic sleeve. On the other hand, if the mechanism of the tap were not defective, then the only other reason for the failure had to be a weakness of the plastic itself. The control knob was sent to a plastics expert in a firm of international repute and he said that the material used was a thermo-setting resin widely used for household electrical fittings. It had high impact strength but was well known for brittleness and could very definitely not perform the task required of it in this knob. The plastic would crumble, as it did. He also reported that manufacturers had recognised this problem and had changed to using glass-reinforced nylon for such sleeves, thus eliminating this type of failure.

It is indeed remarkable that after three years and eight replacements of broken control knobs the housewife should have been blamed for using 'too much force', without being given knobs which would have stood up to normal use.

Case History 2: Accidental Fatal Overdose of Drugs, Self-administered

Coroner's Verdict and Cause of Death
Death from respiratory failure due to soporific poisoning accidentally self-administered.

The deceased was the twenty-year-old daughter of a chartered surveyor and the wife of a salesman. At the time of death she had been married four months and had known her husband for nine months. They had lived in that flat for seven months.

Her husband said that since moving to Bristol she had been very depressed and was receiving treatment at a local hospital. At 8.30 a.m. on Tuesday he left for work and the deceased was up, though not dressed, and waved goodbye to him. In view of her condition she was in reasonably good spirits and gave no indication of anything being wrong. At 6.30 p.m. the husband returned home and saw the post still unopened. His wife was lying in bed in her nightclothes with her head resting on a low bed-side table. As he lifted her back into bed he realised something was seriously wrong, and sent for an ambulance.

There were five bottles of tablets, one of which was empty, on the table by the bed. The husband knew that the empty one should have contained eight sodium amytal tablets. She had been prescribed

fourteen of these the Saturday before and would have taken two each
night since. The other bottles contained anti-depressant medicines.

It would appear that she went back to bed after her husband left.
A note to him lying on a box containing Christmas cards was
identified as being in his wife's handwriting. He said the note must have
been written after he left home. There was also a note to her parents
in the typewriter. It was unfinished. The notes read as follows:

To [husband's name] — my only love, please stay by me. I need your
love so much, I really do.
I love you, there is no doubt about that, its because of that I am
having a longer lie-in than usual in these parts. I love you honey
too much for my own good.

Dearest Mum and Dad, I feel a little sleepy and so I have gone to
bed for a while. I love you both more than any words could ever
say, and my [husband's name] doesn't deserve a silly little girl
like me, he needs a woman to give him good food. I am sick in my
mind, but can't give him the wife he needs. I wish he was here
now to see what a slut I am.
I have just seen the milkman come round. I wish I knew
the co—.

The police arrived at 7.05 p.m.

Her father said that until eighteen months ago she was normal in
every respect, enjoying the company of both sexes, going to dances,
riding in the New Forest, and generally enjoying life. At one time she
intended looking after ponies for a gentleman and was very disappointed
when that fell through. Following this she suffered from bouts of
depression and at Christmas was discharged from a hospital after three
months' psychiatric treatment. The treatment, however, did not improve
her depression. She then went to the North Country for a holiday and
it was there she was prescribed various drugs, including tranquillisers
and sleeping tablets. One of the tablets prescribed had to be taken with
great care because of its possible effect on the other tablets she might
be taking or certain foods. Her father stressed that she was irresponsible
in the way in which she would take her tablets. Perhaps as she had taken
them for so long they were not having the desired effect. She
experienced great difficulty in getting to sleep at night and would still
be writing letters at 3.00 a.m. Sometimes she fell asleep while writing
and tailed off into a scribble. Her parents had received a number of

letters from her just prior to her death. She was looking forward to a visit from them during the Christmas holidays. She had no financial, health or domestic worries and never intimated in any way that she might take her own life.

The general practitioner stated that the deceased had been in his care for six months, during which time she had been treated for severe depression with anti-depressants and sleeping tablets. She always had a regular supply but in small quantities as a precaution against her taking an overdose. He had last prescribed for her on the Saturday before her death. (This was when she received the fourteen sodium amytal capsules referred to by the husband during his evidence.) The pathologist who carried out the post mortem said that the following drugs were found in the body:

Parnate (tranylcypromine)
Valium (diazepam)
Mysoline (primidone)
Distalgesic (dextropropoxyphene and paracetamol)
Barbiturate

Comments

The notes left by the deceased are strongly suggestive of suicidal intent, as is the presumed consumption of six capsules of sodium amytal at one time. Against this is the fact that she had chosen not to take all the tablets from any one of the other bottles which were also within her reach. There also did not appear to be any motive for suicide. It appears that the coroner considered all these possibilities and gave the deceased and her relatives the benefit of any doubt by compassionately returning the verdict of accidental death.

This case illustrates the pharmacological confusion which can arise from the widely accepted and widely practised but nevertheless haphazard drug therapy in psychiatric disorder. This confusion provided the means for her death. The tablet which the father said in evidence had to be taken 'with great care because of its possible effects on the other tablets she might be taking or certain foods' was the monamine oxidase inhibiting group of anti-depressants of which Parnate (tranyl-cypromine), which was present in her body, is a prime example. It is well known that these drugs interact with certain foods such as cheese, Bovril, Marmite, broad beans, yoghurt and alcohol to cause dangerous side effects. These drugs also potentiate the effects of barbiturates so that even a dose which should not prove fatal could nevertheless lead to death. Sodium amytal is a barbiturate and, in the presence of Parnate, the six capsules which she took could have been the chief factor in causing death. Furthermore, the drug Primidone, also found inside her, is changed to barbiturate in the body. It is used to control epilepsy, though there is no evidence that she suffered from it. Her father stressed her irresponsibility in the way she took tablets but it is pertinent to ask whether a person in a disturbed state of mind should be considered capable of remembering the dangers of complicated drug interactions when taking many different kinds of tablets.

Case History 3: Accidental Tissue Bonding by an Adhesive, Fixing Hand in Clenched Position

At about 7 p.m. one evening, I attended to a boy of seventeen who came to the Accident Department in Bath with the fingers and thumb of one hand firmly fixed in a tightly clenched position, following the rupture, a short time earlier, of a small tube of Loctite Super Glue 3, a cyanoacrylate adhesive, in his palm. He had had the tube for some time and had rolled up the lower empty part like a toothpaste tube. It had then proved difficult to squeeze out the contents while fixing a model because the glue had dried on the nozzle. When he therefore firmly squeezed it in his palm, the tube burst where weakened by the rolling and the glue smeared his hand. The tube fell out as he opened his fingers and then, as he closed them again, the adhesive set. In a few seconds his fingers and thumb were fixed. Immediately it had happened he had boiled a kettle and washed the hand in water as hot as he could bear. As the adhesive bond continued to harden, he came to the hospital in a neighbour's car.

There was no information available on what to do to release his fingers. The only address on the tube was one in Ohio, USA. I telephoned a personal friend, an industrial expert in resins, who advised that solvents used for those adhesives would not do for this glue and in any case they would harm the skin. The doctors in the regional plastic surgery unit were also unable to help. Attempts to lift the hardened adhesive off the skin caused pain. As there appeared to be no immediate danger to life or limb, it was decided to admit him to a ward for observation overnight.

At 3 a.m. in the morning the bond released itself. The boy told me later that he felt his palm 'filling with sweat' (it was a very warm night), just before the fingers released themselves. They had been bonded for a total of about eight hours. It seemed to me that sweat collected under the adhesive and lifted it off the skin. From the strength and manner of the bond it appeared highly unlikely that any more persistent or copious lavage would significantly have shortened the time before release.

Comments

Two important considerations arise from this experience.

1. Owing to the free availability of this product and its wide advertising, a real hazard could exist for toddlers who may get hold of a tube, in spite of the warning on it to keep it away from children. If a child bit through a tube and smeared the contents on the lips and nose, an immediate bond would form with possible risk of suffocation. It seems that quick release of the lips would be impossible without the use of a knife. Death could occur quickly before medical help could be obtained. I have since learned that the manufacturers recommend copious lavage with warm water and peeling the glue off the skin. In this case, however, such action was not effective. I have been unable to confirm any certain method of quick release, and this is quite understandable as the glue appears to be very efficient.

2. It is surprising that a substance which can bond living tissue and skin could have been released in this country without any adequate information being first disseminated to medical and para-medical services. Doctors have recently speculated whether surgical separation of bonded tissue might be necessary (*British Medical Journal*, 5 June 1976, letter, no. 6022, 1405 only). A letter from me reporting this case was published in the *British Medical Journal* (24 July 1976, 2, no. 6029, 234 only). This was in turn reported in the *Daily Telegraph* of 29 July 1976, with a statement from the manufacturers that they intended to insert full-page advertisements in medical journals later in the year informing doctors of this product and giving advice, and that they also intended to circulate information to first aid organisations. According to the same report the manufacturer's marketing director in Britain said that American doctors were more conversant with modern adhesives than their colleagues in Britain. Since no one can be informed unless information is made available to them, it is highly likely that American doctors are so well briefed as a result of the activities of statutory bodies in America such as the National Commission on Product Safety, which ensure that new products cannot be marketed before their properties relating to public safety are studied, assessed and publicised.

Case History 4: Fatal Accidental Fall

Coroner's Verdict and Cause of Death
Bronchopneumonia following fractured ribs from an accidental fall.

The deceased was the seventy-three-year-old wife of a retired ware-houseman and lived with her husband in a terraced house in an older part of the city. She was active though her general health was not very good. She became breathless at times and had occasional giddy spells. Her hearing was good but her eyesight was poor even though she wore glasses.

According to evidence given by the husband at the inquest, he went down to the basement to get some coal. The basement was reached by a staircase which had a sharp turn at the bottom. They were both accustomed to the stairs, as they had lived there for twenty-five years. She followed him down and he had reached the bottom and was about to go along the passageway when he heard her shout and at the same time heard her falling. He looked back and saw her lying at the bottom of the stairs. He helped her up and suggested she went to bed for a while, which she did, but was soon up and about although obviously in pain. She went to bed early that evening and the next morning her husband contacted their general practitioner. As a result she was taken to hospital.

In hospital she was found to have fractures of the left ninth rib and right knee cap. The following day she was given a general anaesthetic for an operation on the right knee, took a long time to come round, and was found to have a weakness of the left side of the body. The possibility of a brain tumour was considered and she was taken to a nearby neurosurgical unit, where a special x-ray of the brain excluded it. A stroke was therefore diagnosed and by 7 March she had developed paralysis of one side of her body and, though conscious, was unable to speak. On 5 April she developed an infection in the lung and died ten days later. A post-mortem revealed hardening of the arteries of the brain, a fractured rib and severe pneumonia of both lungs. A verdict of accidental death was returned.

Some months later, allowing time for the husband to become reconciled to the loss of his wife, a doctor and a nurse from the Medical Research Division of the Health Education Council visited him to investigate the accident. The husband was a friendly old man of about seventy years who appeared quite ready to talk about his wife's accident.

On the day of the accident his wife had, as usual, cooked a midday meal of meat and vegetables on the gas stove in their tiny kitchen, which was not much more than a passage approximately 6 feet by 4 feet, with a door at each end and no window. (There was also a flueless Coniston gas water heater installed, although there was no ventilation: the South Western Gas Board had refused to install their usual gas water heater because of this.) After eating, they did the washing up and, while he went to the garden, she washed some clothes. She used the earthenware sink, as she only had some stockings and underwear, and for these she used hot water from the gas water heater. She had finished when he came back inside. He went down to the basement to get some coal and she followed him down the stairs carrying the washing in a plastic bowl. She intended hanging the clothes in the garden, which was reached through the basement. He had reached the basement passage when he heard a bump as his wife fell. The events following this were as stated at the inquest (given above), except that she had complained of a severe headache during that evening.

The staircase was lit by an electric light. Each tread had a piece of rather worn linoleum on it. The danger point appeared to be at the turn of the stairs where the upper handrail on the left stopped and the next three steps came to a point on that side. On enquiry whether the woman had had any similar accident before, he at first said no but then remembered his wife's diary, which she had apparently kept regularly ever since he had first met her over fifty years before. He produced the latest diary and casual inspection revealed that two recent similar falls which did not require treatment had been recorded. Following this interview, it was decided to return later to study the kitchen environment in relation to the function of the gas water heater. This was done some days later.

The test consisted of running the heater and estimating the carbon monoxide and carbon dioxide in the waste gases at the exit on the top of the heater, where they were discharged into the room. A similar test was done in the room atmosphere at head height near the sink. The results of the tests showed that the concentration of carbon monoxide in the room atmosphere was 50 parts per million after 11 minutes, 250 parts per million after 22 minutes, and 400 parts per million after 29 minutes. The maximum permissible concentration of carbon monoxide in an industrial working environment is 50 parts per million. This speaks for itself. For the rate of increase found in the kitchen, it is predicted that after one hour's continual running of the heater (which could be possible with this type of heater on wash day), the carbon monoxide level in the room, with both doors shut, would rise to about 1000 parts per million. If a person were engaged in light work in the kitchen while using the heater, the level of carboxyhaemo-globin in the blood could rise to 12 per cent in 15 minutes (the normal level is 1 to 5 per cent).[1] Continued exposure for longer periods would result in correspondingly higher levels.

Comments

Although this was a case of an elderly woman who fell down a staircase which had several hazardous features, and although this was the prin-cipal concern at the inquest, none of the hazards were mentioned. More detailed subsequent investigation of the antecedent events showed that the woman had spent at least three hours and probably more, prior to the fall, in a kitchen atmosphere which contained a dangerous gas heater installation. Since the heater was not examined soon after the fall and because no blood was examined for carbon monoxide, it is impossible to be sure that she was suffering from the ill effects of carbon monoxide inhalation. However it seems highly likely that this may have been a contributory factor in the fall.

This case is a good example of how accidents are often caused by the interaction of a number of factors. It also illustrates the stifling effect which the term 'accidental death', with its implication of inevitability, can have in the investigation of an accident.

Notes

1.   W. H. Forbes, F. Sargent and F. J. W. Roughton (1945), 'The rate of carbon monoxide uptake by normal men', *American Journal of Physiology*, Vol. 143, p. 594.

2 ACCOUNTING FOR ACCIDENTAL INJURY IN CHILDHOOD

M. Calnan and M. Wadsworth

Introduction

Childhood accidents have always been seen as an important area for study, although perhaps in proportion to incidence it has been an under-investigated subject. Recent concern about child 'abuse' or non-accidental injury to children has stimulated further work, and this paper presents a selective review of how accidents are studied by epidemiologists, psychologists and sociologists, and suggests the need for a change in emphasis. It does not consider the psychological and psycho-physiological studies of the effects of clumsiness and poor motor coordination.

Incidence

Mortality in childhood because of accidental injury forms an important proportion of all childhood deaths during the ages of 1 to 4 years. It is true that 'in 1932 . . . approximately 6% of all deaths in England and Wales in the 1-4 years old age group were due to accidents' and that 'by 1972 the proportion was 24%' (Office of Health Economics, 1975), yet as the Office of Health Economics points out, the actual number of deaths has been going down.[1]

Morbidity rates are more difficult to discover. The large longitudinal studies which have each followed up a population of children over a period of years are the obvious sources of data, but they show remarkable differences in rates. In the Newcastle study Miller and his colleagues (1960) report 'an incidence of about 1 accident per child' (p. 138) by the age of five years, but in the National Survey of Health and Development Douglas and Blomfield (1958) found that 24.1 per cent of children had been injured by this age. Of the 581 first-born offspring of the National Survey cohort so far investigated,[2] 40.5 per cent had been injured by the age of four years. On the other hand the National Child Development Study found that by eleven years of age 28.6 per cent of children had been accidentally injured (C. Peckham, 1976, personal communication).

Few population figures are available about how many children suffer more than one accident, but in the study of National Survey offspring

7.1 per cent had been injured more than once by age four years and had received medical treatment on each occasion. We can find no published information about differences in rates of accidental injury as between siblings in the same family, but it seems to be a subject in need of investigation.

Evidently the definition of an accident is far from clear, and some of the difficulties that are involved are now discussed.

Review and Summary of Explanations

One of the greatest difficulties in studying accidental injury is the selection of the study population, and it is especially difficult in the case of childhood injuries, since the universe of variables to be investigated is usually delineated only by age. It is practically impossible to know how much 'at risk' children are from accidents. Whereas it can be said of pilots that, for example, hours of flying and numbers of particular manoeuvres can be seen as quantifying 'at-riskness', in studies of children there is no comparable measure. Restricting studies to particular *types* of childhood accidents is of little help since amounts of bicycle riding, or standing within the vicinity of cookers or fires is unlikely to be accurately assessed. As a consequence most studies have taken a sample or series of patients attending an accident and emergency department, and asked the injured person or parent for details of the accident, and for a description of whatever aspects of their lives the investigator thinks may be relevant. Some studies have taken a sample of patients and matched them with a non-injured control group (e.g. Wehrle, Day, Whalen, Fitzgerald and Harris, 1960), others have been concerned only with the injured population itself (e.g. Husband and Hinton, 1972).

Studies of accidents to children have usually looked for predisposing features in three particular aspects of the child's environment or way of life; first the physical environment itself. As well as dangers associated with faulty electrical equipment, open fires and cooking, overcrowded home circumstances and the absence of protected play space have also been implicated as predisposing factors, the latter, for example, in road accidents (Backett and Johnston, 1959). Similarly, in a study of accidental poisoning McKendrick (1960) found that the major contributory factor was that the poison had been kept in an 'inappropriate place'. The second environmental feature concerns the dangers inevitably associated with normal physical development. Rowntree (1950) noted that 'when the children were beginning to sit up, to grab objects within reach and especially when they were beginning to walk, they were exposed to many more risks, whatever kind of home they were living in'. More recently Jackson, Walker and Wynne (1968) concluded that 'the child is poisoned because of his lack of experience, his inquisitiveness, and his inability to understand the consequences of his actions'. Inevitably, therefore, the third environmental feature is parental supervision, since in all the circumstances already mentioned it could generally be concluded, although perhaps not so readily in some individual cases, that more rigorous parental supervision could have avoided the accident. In their study of burns and scalded children Shelmerdine and Rigby (1974) noted that the lack of parental supervision was the crucial predisposing factor, and Mitchell (1967) concluded that 'children are more likely to be seriously burned in homes where economic privation or parental disharmony have impaired the quality of maternal care'.

More recently accident studies have tended to go beyond these three environmental or way-of-life features of the children and their parents, and have seen the accident as a reflection of 'something going wrong' in personal relationships, either between the child and his siblings or parents, or between the parents. Possibly this development of the subject areas searched for explanation has come not only from the conclusions about parental supervision, but also, by example, from the better controlled (in research terms) studies of accidents, where the concept of at-riskness is quantifiable. For example, studies of pilots have compared those who have accidents or near-accidents or who suddenly develop flying phobia, which is associated with an increased likelihood of accident, with those who do not. In their study of flying phobia Daly, Aitken and Rosenthal (1970) found that 'a striking feature in many cases was a similarity of social precipitance . . . symptoms were often preceded and accompanied by psycho-social stress, such as sexual or marital problems'.

The many studies that look for a specific set of social or psychological personal circumstances 'behind' accidents have done so from various points of view. Some investigators, for example Brenner (1964), favour psychoanalytic interpretation, and seek explanation of accidents as symbolic 'acting out' behaviour. He explained that a lady driver involved in a shunt type of accident was in fact demonstrating symbolically against her husband's maltreatment of her, and against his inability to satisy her sexually by 'having a man bang into her tail'. Mitchell (1967) felt that 'the ingestion of a poisonous household chemical so far from being a chance act of an aimlessly exploring child, is often a deliberate attempt to provoke or punish the parent.'

Other investigations have looked for a particular personality trait in the child. Baltimore and Meyer (1969) for example, found that the cause of poisoning in fifty-two children when compared with controls lay not in such environmental factors as storage of medicine, but rather in the higher incidence of extroversion, impulsiveness, daringness and exaggerated oral tendencies amongst the injured group. And Mellinger and Manheimer (1967) argued that a child's ability to cope with hazards was impaired by maladjustment.

Some studies have looked much more to personal relationships as a source of explanation, than to the supposedly stable traits of personality measures. These explanations can be seen as having two sorts of emphasis. Some of them conclude that the child's usual mode of relationships with his family is of the greatest importance, whilst others implicate a particular set of circumstances that took place at the time of the accident. Marcus and his colleagues (1964), for example, found that the child's

> closeness and identification with the family appear to be weaker than in our control groups. The family pattern is disturbed and contributed to the child's insecurity and anxiety. The accident pattern appears to be a syndrome indicative of emotional disturbance within an individual who relies on action as his chief defensive mechanism against anxiety.

Wight (1969) concluded that some kinds of accidents were associated with a low level of mothers' responsiveness to the baby's behaviour, which he took to be a sensitive indicator of mother-baby interaction. On the other hand, Sobel (1971) felt that the most important elements in the explanation of why children were poisoned lay 'not in the realm of home safety, intelligence or motor precocity, not in the struggle for power or childhood mental disturbance, but in environmental instability, parental disorder and breakdown of marriage'. This view, which rests on the assumption that the child's behaviour is altered when family relationships are unhappy, may be summarised in the conclusions of Meyer and his colleagues (1963) who found that

> . . . each child was caught in a circumstantial web involving developmental, family and environmental hazard drawing them closer to injury. The superimposed 'climate of stress' within many homes provided further difficulty for the child, often distracting parents from their child's predicament.

With this trend towards the interpretation of childhood accidents as signs of 'something wrong' in family relationships, it is not surprising that researchers have begun to suggest that there may sometimes be little difference between the circumstances which produce non-accidental injury and those leading to accidental injury. For instance, Martin (1970) suggests that burns may sometimes be symptoms of parental hostility towards their young children and more recently evidence of child abuse by non-accidental poisoning has been presented by Rogers and his colleagues (1976).

Discussion

Before putting forward our proposals for ways of going about studying accidents, we think it necessary to make a number of critical observations in general about the published studies.

First, it is evident that the wide range of sampling techniques used make comparison of studies difficult. The research which uses clinic samples, even with controls, will have little real knowledge of the representativeness of attenders. It can be argued that all those with serious injuries go for medical treatment, and that as seriousness decreases so does the likelihood of using medical care. However, there are reasons to believe that this is not the case, and that the less seriously injured, who in fact make up the greater part of accident and emergency treatment work, are not representative of all those with less serious injuries. Some children will be taken for treatment, more or less regardless of seriousness of injury, by childminders and play supervisors, as a measure of protection against possible later legal proceedings. Those who are injured at friends' houses, as an unexpectedly high proportion of children suspected of being poisoned were in one study (Calnan, 1975), are also more likely to be taken for medical treatment as a precautionary measure. At the hospital itself some treatment, for example of head injuries or poisoning, will be given in case a real injury has occurred, although in some cases it will ultimately turn out to have been unnecessary. Admission to hospital may also be just as much a function of non-medical as medical factors, and it is known that some groups in the population seek treatment less readily than others (see McKinlay (1972) for a review). Under-utilisation of medical services by families in the lower socio-economic groups is well documented, and Calnan, Dale and de Fonseka (1976), in a study of children with suspected poisoning, found that such families were more likely to delay seeking care until very clear evidence of poisoning occurred, whereas upper social class parents tended to contact the services immediately poisoning was suspected. This evidence is congruent with previous work which has shown a greater use of the preventive health services by middle-class groups (Bloor and Gill, 1972).

Second, it seems unlikely that the home physical environment *per se* plays a particularly important role in the majority of childhood accidents. Although it could be argued that in relation to some types of accident the home environment is now safer for children (e.g. open fires are fewer), we do not in fact see a great reduction in numbers of injuries, and of course the environment outside the home is now as hazardous as ever. Recent work on the effects on family relationships of living in a poor home environment concluded that 'crowded conditions seldom have any consequences and even when they do the effects are very modest' (Booth and Edwards, 1976). If environmental factors were of the greatest importance, then we would expect to find a high rate of injury amongst all the children of families living in such circumstances, but this seems not to have been investigated. In fact, those workers who stressed the importance of environmental factors also speak at the least of the importance of parental care and super-vision, if not of relationships and interactions between the mother and the child.

Our final comment concerns findings about family stress and upheaval of relationships. Evaluation of such work is particularly difficult since there are few data about the prevalence of 'stressful events'. The question has to be raised as to why in stressful families apparently not all children suffer accidents. It could be that they do, and that the accidents vary in severity, or that mothers have thresh-holds of consulting medical care that differ as between children. There is evidence of differential treatment of children, and certainly it seems that 'child abuse' often concerns only one of the children in a family. These kinds of findings subscribe equally well to the hypotheses about the function of parents' and childrens' personalities in the incidence of accidents, as to that of 'stressful events'.

Thus, whilst we see the balance of evidence to be in favour of explanations that take into account the family's personal and social circumstances, we feel that the published work has not taken sufficient note of some factors, for example the effects of sampling procedures, nor has yet been broad enough in concept really to investigate the phenomenon.

Proposals

We suggest that certain new dimensions are required. In order to understand fully the effects of any factor on childhood injury it is necessary to see whether this factor has the same effect on all the children in the family or not, since factors which apparently act selectively, affecting only one child, would indicate that research should be more child-centred. As Rutter (1976) recently noted 'it is no new observation that children differ in their responses to stress situations but until recent years surprisingly little attention has been paid to this side of parent-child interaction . . .' (p. 182). This, therefore, argues for a whole-family study of injury, which would take into account not only the home physical environment but also family relationships. This would aim to study all accidental injury, from very minor to very serious, and would be a source of information on differential parental treatment of children and use of care services.

Such studies would also be necessary for investigating repeated injuries occurring to the same child, which is an aspect of childhood injury which is only just beginning to be investigated, and one which should shed much light on findings that relate parent-child relationships to the incidence of childhood injury. Studies of repeated accidents will also involve investigating what happens in families *after* accidents have occurred, a subject which has received surprisingly little attention. It is reasonable to suppose that after an accident those involved will think it over and try to account for it. Many mothers will feel guilt, especially if there are visible signs or effects remaining after some time. Wolff (1969) found that mothers of burnt children who lived even under conditions where accident prevention might be impossible, felt 'profoundly guilty and lose their confidence in themselves as good mothers' (p. 64). Calnan (1975) found that the majority of mothers of children thought to have been poisoned attributed blame to themselves in not putting the toxic substances out of reach and locked away. This personal search for a cause, and a conclusion of self-blame happens not only after accidents but also in cases of mental handicap, as the parental accounts edited by Cooper and Henderson (1973) vividly show. They found that in their search for causes of mental handicap parents often blamed childhood accidents. It is therefore necessary to investigate this important area of how parents and children account for accidents, since it should give clues about their subsequent behaviour as well as about their family relationships.

Parents' accounts are not constructed in isolation. There will be a variety of influences, including other family members and people considered to have significant and appropriate knowledge, amongst them the doctor. Wolff (1969) draws attention to the fact that not only do guilt feelings occur anyway, but often the circumstances of treatment exacerbate and reinforce such feelings. She notes (p. 64) that:

> . . . doctors and nurses tend to attribute the accident to carelessness especially when, as is so often the case, the family belongs to that socio-economic group with which middle class hospital staff have least in common. Their critical attitudes and their inability to identify with a family tend to reinforce the parents' feelings of guilt and inadequacy.

As a result, effects on later parent-child relationships might well be damaged. In some cases there could be a risk of disturbance following hospitalisation (see e.g. Douglas, 1975), especially if there was a relationship between the accident happening and disturbed child-parent relationships. The study of the first born offspring of the National Survey of Health and Development shows that burnt children were significantly more likely to have mothers who reported after the event that they felt emotionally cool towards the child, who felt worried about 'going wrong' in bringing up this child, who felt worried about him coping with school and worried about their own management of discipline. Although it cannot be known whether these mothers felt like this before the accident or became so as a result of it, the findings still argue for longer term follow-up rather than episodic studies of injured children and their families.

We feel that studies which set out to look at repeated accidents and accidental injury within sibships as we have suggested here, would go some way to answering particularly important questions about how factors, already shown to be or suspected of being related to injury, actually operate. In doing so they will help to solve some of the sampling problems we have noted as characteristic of studies of child-hood accidents, by focusing attention not so much on the accident itself, but on, say, particular kinds of maternal/child relationships or particular treatment experiences, and then looking at the incidence of injury in relation to them. Obviously the sort of investigation best suited to these tasks is a longitudinal study; the three current national longitudinal studies[3] should be able to provide information on incidence rates both of accidents and of some kinds of events generally expected to be stressful, and to investigate how these relate to one another and to the home physical environment. Smaller follow-up studies, perhaps of particular groups of the national cohort members, of smaller populations (such as the study by Richards, 1974) and of complete families, should be a source of more intensive data, such as parents' own accounts of why accidents happened and of treatment experience.

We think that rather than continuing to study childhood accidents by taking a sample of patients attending an Accident and Emergency department and looking for 'causes' amongst recalled data selected by the investigators, it would now be more fruitful to look at accidents in a broader way. Accidents should be investigated in their real family social context, and over time, with a recognition that the parent's and the injured child's ways of accounting for the accident form an essential part of understanding why the accident happened to this child and a basis for asking whether it may happen again.

Notes

1. In 1972 the actual number of deaths by accidental injury under the age of five years was 696.
2. In a study which is being carried out by the second author.
3. These are the National Survey of Health and Development which has regularly studied a cohort of 5362 children from birth in 1946 to the present (Douglas, Ross and Simpson, 1969), the National Child Development Study which has regularly studied a cohort of 16,000 children from birth in 1958 to the present (Davie, Butler and Goldstein, 1972) and the Child Health and Education in the Seventies study of 18,000 children born in 1970 and now being followed up under the direction of Professor N. R. Butler of the Department of Child Health at the University of Bristol.

References

Backett, E. M. and Johnston, A. M. (1959) Social patterns of road accidents to children. *British Medical Journal* 1, 409-13.

Baltimore, C. and Meyer, R. J. (1969) A study of storage, child behavioral traits, and mothers' knowledge of toxicology in 52 poisoned families and 52 comparison families. *Pediatrics* 44, 816-29.

Bloor, M. J. and Gill, D. G. (1972) Screening of the well child: a discussion of some of the problems involved. *Community Medicine*, 129, 135-8.

Booth, A. and Edwards, J. N. (1976) Crowding and family relations. *American Sociological Review*, 41, 308-21.

Brenner, C. (1964) Prapraxes and wit, in *Accident Research* (eds. W. Haddon, E. A. Suchman and D. Klein), pp. 292-5. New York: Harper and Row.

Calnan, M. W. (1975) Sociological Factors in Accidental Child Poisoning. Unpublished MSc thesis, University of Bristol.

Calnan, M. W., Dale, J. W. and de Fonseka, C. P. (1976) Suspected poisoning in children. *Archives of Disease in Childhood* **51**, 180-5.

Cooper, L. and Henderson, R. (1973) *Something Wrong.* London: Arrow Books.

Daly, R. J., Aitken, R. C. B. and Rosenthal, S. V. (1970) Flying phobia: phenomenological study. *Proc. Royal Society of Medicine,* **63**, 14-18.

Davie, R., Butler, N. and Goldstein, H. (1972) *From Birth to Seven.* London: Longman.

Douglas, J. W. B. and Blomfield, J. M. (1958) *Children Under Five.* London: Allen and Unwin.

Douglas, J. W. B., Ross, J. M. and Simpson, H. R. (1968) *All our Future.* London: Peter Davies.

Douglas, J. W. B. (1975) Early hospital admissions and later disturbances of behaviour and learning. *Developmental Medicine and Child Neurology,* **17**, 456-80.

Husband, P. and Hinton, P. E. (1972) Families of children with repeated accidents. *Archives of Disease in Childhood,* **47**, 396-400.

Jackson, R. H., Walker, J. H. and Wynne, N. A. (1968) Circumstances of accidental poisoning in childhood. *British Medical Journal,* **4**, 245-8.

Marcus, I. W., Wilson, W., Kraft, I., Swander, D., Southerland, F. and Schuchofer, E. (1964) in Haddon *et al.* (eds.), op. cit., 313-26.

Martin, H. L. (1970) Antecedents of burns and scalds in children. *British Journal of Medical Psychology,* **43**, 39-47.

McKendrick, T. (1960) Poisoning in childhood. *Archives of Disease in Childhood,* **35**, 127-33.

McKinlay, J. B. (1972) Use of services: an overview. *Journal of Health and Social Behaviour,* **2**, 115-22.

Mellinger, G. D. and Manheimer, D. I. (1967) An exposure-coping model of accident liability among children. *Journal of Health and Social Behaviour,* **8**, 96-106.

Meyer, R. J., Roelofs, H. A., Bluestone, E. J. and Redmond, S. (1963) Accidental injury to the pre-school child. *Journal of Pediatrics,* **63**, 95-105.

Miller, F. J. W., Court, S. D. M., Walton, W. S. and Knox, E. G. (1960) *Growing up in Newcastle-upon-Tyne.* London: OUP.

Mitchell, R. G. (1967) Accidents in childhood. *Developmental Medicine and Child Neurology* **9**, 767-9.

Office of Health Economics (1975) *Accidental Deaths* (OHE Briefing Pamphlet No. 2). London: Office of Health Economics.

Richards, M. P. M. (1974) An ecological study of infant development in an urban setting in Britain. Paper to a Wenner-Gren Symposium at Burg Wartenstein. Mimeo.

Rogers, D., Tripp, J., Bentovim, A., Robinson, A., Berry, D. and Goulding, R. (1976) Non-accidental poisoning: an extended syndrome of child abuse. *British Medical Journal* **1**, 793-6.

Rowntree, G. (1950) Accidents among children under two years of age in Great Britain, *Journal of Hygiene* **48**, 325-37.

Rutter, M. (1976) Parent-child separation: psychological effects on the children, in *Early Experience: Myth and Evidence* (eds. Ann M. Clarke and A. D. B. Clarke). London: Open Books.

Shelmerdine, H. R. and Rigby, M. J. (1974) Home accident survey. *Health and Social Services Journal* **74**, 542-3.

,Sobel, R. (1971) Psychiatric implications of child poisoning. *Pediatric Clinics of North America* 17, 653-6.

Wehrle, P. F., Day, P. A., Whalen, J. P., Fitzgerald, J. W. and Harris, V. G. (1960) Epidemiology of accidental child poisoning in an urban population. *American Journal of Public Health* 50, 1925-33.

Wight, B. W. (1969) The control of child-environment interaction: a conceptual approach to accident occurrence. *Pediatrics* 44, 799-805

Wolff, S. (1969) *Children Under Stress.* London: Allen Lane, The Penguin Press.

3 HUMAN BEHAVIOUR IN DOMESTIC FIRES

J. Breaux, D. Canter and J. Sime

The reader may wonder, on seeing the above title, what there is to be said about human behaviour in fires. The obvious interpretation of our title would seem to be that our paper deals with human behaviour leading to fires. It is less likely that one would, at first glance, assume the title to mean human behaviour during fires, since the possible variations in behaviour at that time might seem very limited. This is, to a large extent, due to the fact that many people have never directly experienced a fire in the home. What they have heard or read about them in newspapers, coupled with commonsense, leads them to expect that human behaviour during a fire should be relatively straightforward, with but few alternatives or complications. This paper attempts to indicate the true complexity of human behaviour in a fire situation and point to those factors integral to such an understanding. A general model is presented which indicates possible behaviour sequences and gives some idea of how our current knowledge fits together.

There are several reasons why this paper focuses on subsequent aspects of the accident process rather than on the original cause of the fire (cf. also Canter and Matthews, 1976). First, even granted vast funds to eliminate the causes, we cannot expect the phenomenon of fires to disappear. It is likely that, as ever more is spent in the attempt to eliminate fires, an asymptote will be reached beyond which further investment will in effect constitute a loss. Second, such an approach would be unlikely to take full account of the role of motivation in the causation of fires. Our research is starting to indicate instances in which it seems that accidents were 'allowed to happen', this having nothing to do with financial gain or deliberate fire setting. These often concern 'acts of omission' as opposed to 'acts of commission'. Others (e.g. Hansbrough, 1961) have noted similar peculiarities in the 'accident' process which at times yield positive outcomes for those concerned. Third, since fires do occur, effort should be expended on minimising negative consequences. What is it about certain fires, buildings, and the people involved which culminates in death and injury? The answers are not always apparent. Stapelfeldt (1975) notes of a discothèque fire, for example, 'A young woman carrying a baby and a man with one leg in plaster who had been quite close to the point where the fire started escaped unhurt whereas those suffering from smoke poisoning and those who later died had been much closer to the exits' (p. 10). This type of paradox occurs quite frequently. Research by the Fire Research Unit at the University of Surrey has already indicated a number of such paradoxes. Given that building design codes aim for a situation in which occupants can leave a structure unaided and by their own efforts in the event of fire, the study of why some people do well and others worse in effect constitutes the study of an accident within an accident. It is, in fact, this compounding of events and their consequences which we will attempt to delineate. The implication here is that the danger of fire to people is not always inherent in its *ignition* but in the way it *develops* and how that relates to human behaviour – the so-called 'secondary' effects according to Zwingmann (1971).

GENERAL BACKGROUND

Recently, Canter and Matthews (1976) have outlined an approach to the study of behaviour in fires which, apart from indicating the need for new information, given rapid architectural change, points to alternative ways of viewing the problem. We note, for example, a shift in the thinking which has tended to regard behaviour in fires as essentially dichotomous in outcome: escape versus no escape (e.g. Phillips, 1975). It is replaced by a scheme which is sensitive to such options as seeking refuge within the building, putting out the fire, warning others, and otherwise coping. In addition to noting that building regulations do not adequately inform people of the desired sequence of behaviour, given various possible courses of action, it demonstrates that such regulations are often based on false assumptions which correspond poorly to real events (e.g. the unit width and its relation to movement).[1] It is, in this respect, primarily the work of Pauls (1971a, 1971b) and by implication, Melinek (1975), which points to the contradiction inherent in that which is expected and what we actually observe during evacuations. It is not that one expects perfection in the formulae underlying evacuation-time predictions but, as noted by Pauls (1974), these are often out by 50 to 100 per cent. This, however, is but one example of what are often inappropriate assumptions concerning human behaviour.

Other writers take for granted (or imply) a high potential for 'panic' behaviour (Melinek, 1975; Murray and Finch, 1975). They obtain little support for such views, given existing evidence (Quarantelli, 1973; Wood, 1972) which suggests that bizarre and extreme behaviour is the exception rather than the rule (or even the trend). Clearly, we will have to amend our ideas of what constitutes true panic. It is conceivable that what, in a *post hoc* analysis, appears to be the end result of panic (stampeding ending in trampling, for example) is the undesirable outcome of rational behaviour under marked constraints. But no matter how logically we might reduce the situations or indicate their relative infrequency, that one such event might occur and not have been provided for is something we all wish to avoid.

The above examples, pointing as they do to the implications of new information, suggest potential problems as to how one implements knowledge. Since we are trying to relate behaviour to certain environments and regulations associated with these, it is likely that some of our findings will indicate, like Pauls', that we cannot always count on optimal responses to help guarantee the safety of building occupants. Thus egress formulae which assume rates of 40 to 45 individuals per minute per unit width are overly optimistic, given what we know from realistic drills and evacuations. It may, for example, be possible to remedy this situation by teaching people how to behave more efficiently, thereby bringing their actions more in line with flow expectations (e.g. sensitise them to the personal buffer zone phenomenon).[2] On the other hand, we can recommend alternative evacuation procedures or the implementation of different building features (e.g. certain types of refuge areas) which could make up what was lost through unrealistic assumptions. In any event, we are, given such a finding, working towards an improvement in the safety of the system by expending more effort and resources on it.

However, findings such as Quarantelli's (1973) and Wood's (1972) concerning the low incidence of panic can, if taken to their logical conclusion, imply that we might be overly cautious with regard to certain outcomes. In the face of such evidence, one could reasonably conclude that, by eliminating certain redundant or unnecessary safeguards, the system could be made more efficient while leaving the safety factor unaffected. At this level one could invoke cost-benefit analyses to help resolve the issue. It is always easier to recommend changes which are aimed at improving the short or long range safety of people. This we can do and may go so far, if there are sufficient funds, as to 'over provide' (Canter and Matthews, 1976) for most contingencies, thereby assuring ourselves that everything reasonably possible was done. It is considerably more difficult to suggest an improvement in the efficiency of a system deriving from the removal of a safeguard which might apply to but one in 5,000 cases.

Other outcomes are less problematic. It is possible that certain attitudes concerning peoples' behaviour may be inappropriate. It is often assumed, for example, that people lend credence to and react immediately upon hearing alarms and warning signals. Major civil defence systems operate on this assumption (e.g. Williams, 1964). It is even taken for granted in certain cases that warning systems could be activated at the last moment in the belief that the desired reaction will be immediate (Joyce, 1972). Previous research has shown this not to be the case (e.g. Mack and Baker, 1961; Fritz, 1972; Burch, 1971). In fact, even on those occasions when sirens or alarms have signalled extremely dangerous events (e.g. potential nuclear exchanges), pre-scribed reaction has not only been delayed, if it occurred at all, but the signal itself received with low credibility (Williams, 1964). It might be that planners will have to think in terms of time lag when assessing these systems, or alternatively, more effective systems may need to be developed. Melinek (1975) notes, for example, that where discrepancies exist between calculated and observed evacuation times, the equations yield underestimates (approximately two minutes irrespective of the number of floors to be evacuated). This he attributes to a general response delay although it should be stressed that these data are based on pre-announced evacuation drills. Pauls' (1971a) research implies a considerably more erratic pattern of discrepancies between calculations and observations.

Even though such a finding can have policy implications, it represents in the first instance evidence against the view that people respond as expected upon hearing alarms. Consequently, it poses the qustion 'Why?' It is here that, when resolved, such variables as signal credibility and the role of others in the interpretation process contribute to an overall model of behaviour in such situations.

The three general outcomes outlined above (safety improvement, efficiency improvement and an understanding of behaviour) are, of course, not mutually exclusive and do overlap. In the final analysis any finding will increase our knowledge of such events and contribute towards an improvement of the system.

In the next section a general model is presented which will (a) give some idea of how our current knowledge fits together, and (b) indicate possible behaviour sequences. Occasionally points from this model will be illustrated with reference to data the Fire Research Unit has obtained in the course of its research. At times the reader may be in doubt as to how a specific aspect of the model applies to the domestic situation. Occasionally such apprehension may be justified in so far as an attempt has been made to incorporate and summarise all knowledge concerning human behaviour in fires. It should be further appreciated that although the labels 'domestic' and 'non-domestic' appear to describe discrete categories of fires, behavioural communalities exist across both. As noted below, numerous domestic fires take place in buildings not usually associated with the concept 'home'. For this reason factors like expected group evacuation time and the role of others can be relevant in the case of high-rise and multi-occupancy residential blocks.

PRELIMINARY MODEL OF BEHAVIOURAL FACTORS

Referring to Figure 1, one notes that the model centres around three process states: (1) recognition/interpretation, (2) behaviour (action/ no action), and (3) outcomes (evaluation and long-term effects). Each of these is the result of factors which are represented as input variables. Thus at the recognition/interpretation stage, three major inputs (factors immediately arising, past experience and 'current state factors') help in determining how the situation is evaluated. The small circles denote components of each such input. A 'dictionary' is provided below which lists and briefly elaborates upon all aspects of the model. Although the general sequence is indicated by the relative position of the three main stages, certain input components exert influence at more than one stage. In order to illustrate the nature of such relationships a few multiple linkages within the system are indicated by broken lines. Clearly, the model as it now stands is not intended to be exhaustive, and the recent arrival of new information already suggests modifications. Following the elaboration of each main process state, a general summary section listing the relevant findings of the Fire Research Unit to date is included. This is not intended to be a quantitive review; work on that aspect of the research is currently in progress.

Model Dictionary

The model is comprised of three main parts: stages, inputs and components.

A. Stage I: Recognition/Interpretation

This stage represents a process whereby certain information relating to a fire situation is perceived and evaluated.

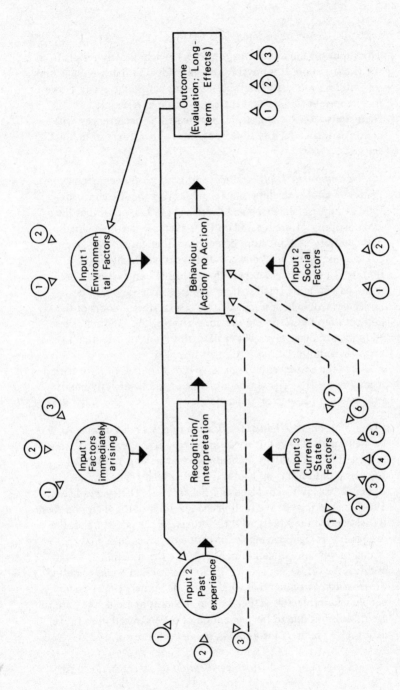

Figure 1. Generalised systems model for human behaviour in fires

Input 1: Factors immediately arising

This input subsumes information (cues) which directly results from the fire situation. It is novel for the individual in that we can assume this information not to have been present before the event. However, it is important to note that these may at times resemble characteristics associated with less threatening occurrences. One can conceive of such factors as deriving from either direct or indirect sources.

(a)   *Component 1: immediately verifiable crisis cues.* Seeing flames or smoke, smelling smoke and hearing the fire constitute valid examples. Globerson and Crossman (1972) report that the great majority of fires (based on USA data) are detected visually, with auditory and olfactory detection trailing far behind. One could argue that a breakdown of fire types would alter this finding. Thus we might expect that in highly compartmentalised areas, detection by smell is more frequent since vapour or gas molecules would be less impeded by cracks around doors or the join between the soffit and the door. Hearing the fire itself is less common although, given better data, this mode of detection may prove to be important in certain settings.

All of the above can be seen to be *direct* sources of information regarding the fire. The sensing of flame or smoke directly implies fire, whether planned or unplanned.

(b)   *Component 2: visual verification of others' behaviour.* As will be mentioned below, this seems important at the level of determining whether a potentially ambiguous situation (e.g. having heard a fire alarm but sensing no fire) is treated as really dangerous. Research has indicated (Mack and Baker, 1961; Darley and Latané, 1968) that in uncertain situations people look to those around them to help define the situation. If the others appear undisturbed, the probability is high, barring the intrusion of direct cues, that the evaluator will also remain calm or redefine the situation as a non-event. However, seeing another person take action seems to define the situation as a potentially real crisis (cf. Turner, 1969) where people take protective action, not on the basis of seeing the harmful agent itself but due to the perception of others' reaction to it, we can speak of indirect information or cues (cf. Breaux, 1975).

(c)   *Component 3: auditory verification of others' actions.* An additional indirect cue has come to our attention quite recently after making detailed observations of a local fire drill (unannounced). There was one person living on the third floor who, upon hearing running — that is, heavy footfalls — defined the drill as a potentially 'real' event. He inferred danger from others' actions. An interesting reaction here was that, upon hearing the alarm, most of those interviewed, with the exception of a small group (the members of which had observed the house warden running in apparent distress), took it to be a drill. The individual who heard running noted that he quickly changed his interpretation and assumed that there could be a fire.

Pauls (1971a) has reported analogous responses to unannounced fire drills. In one instance, 80 per cent of those interviewed interpreted the alarm as signalling a drill or other non-emergency. Interesting in terms of indirect auditory verification was the finding that, although the majority believed the situation to be a drill, the *nervous* delivery of evacuation instructions over a public address system caused two thirds of this group to redefine the event as real. In this case we must assume that a nervous voice implied for the listener that the speaker had direct knowledge of a real hazard.

Input 2: Past experience

This covers past events which could influence a person's evaluation of an alarm or other danger signal.

(a)   *Component 1: number of prior 'false' experiences of a related nature* (fire drills, bomb scares, evacuation drills, etc.). People with a previous history of extensive fire drill involvement can be expected, on hearing an alarm, not to treat it seriously (other things being equal — that is, no additional direct or indirect cues). They probably have habituated to the signal, that is, no longer take it seriously. Thus one case presently being investigated by the Fire Research Unit indicated that several members of a resort staff at first doubted the existence of a fire since they were used to numerous drills during the preceding months.

(b)   *Component 2: previous involvement with extreme situations.* Having been involved in a fire is a case in point. Thus Stahl (1975) has noted that knowledge of an actual fire tends to confirm the fears people have of them. We can expect this to make one more cautious in evaluating initially ambiguous information the next time it happens. Green (1974) reports an analogous effect as regards forest fires.

One can also think of indirect previous involvement, as when someone we know has been involved in a fire or if we read about a terrible incident. It has been suggested (Green, 1974) that since fires accompanied by high fatalities are infrequent, their occurrence has a disproportionate effect on public concern. It may be that the reaction to ambiguous stimuli is more cautious if a few days earlier the press has publicised a nasty occurrence. We might even hypothesise, if this is so, that statistics might indicate a drop in smaller household fires directly following a well-publicised case where numerous deaths occurred.

This proposed effect is analogous to the way in which some people come to re-evaluate bodily sensations during publicised epidemics. What was once quite common often comes to be interpreted in terms of a new causal agent. Thus a mild stomach upset may incorrectly be attributed to influenza. In this case there is a process of relabelling the cause. When a previously unnoticed stimulus takes on greater significance in the detection of some danger one can speak of sensitisation or readjustment (lowering) of the criterion. In this manner fire cues with a high probability of being disregarded could, following a sensitising event, become more salient and lead to immediate investigation (cf. Evans, 1969).

Existing information concerning peoples' reactions to warning systems (Mack and Baker, 1961; Fritz, 1972; Burch, 1971) tells us that few expect the worst to happen. Related to this is the tendency for unknown hazards to be treated with greater caution than known or 'common' ones (Slovic, 1972). We might speculate that if a building were equipped with two types of alarm, one for nuclear radiation warning and the other for conventional fire, assuming both events are perceived as mutually exclusive, the former would be more effective. Fires are common in so far as we have heard much about them. It might be that a more exotic but equally lethal danger has different implications for cue evaluation and behaviour.

(c)   *Component 3: personality characteristics.* At the most basic level it is possible that certain people are overly cautious, whereas others seldom prepare for or expect a crisis. Part of this can be traced to peculiarities in human decision making. A person may see his chances of becoming involved in a fire as lower than they are according to the statistics. One can make an analogy here to a so-called 'Pollyanna' effect in which the probability of an unpleasant event is subjectively underestimated, serving perhaps to raise the threshold at which we evaluate cues as dangerous. Nice events, however, are seen as more likely than they might objectively be (viz. the success of lotteries and pools).

At a different level we have the 'true' personality characteristics. Thus anxiety, dependence and susceptibility to hypochondria supposedly distinguish panic-prone individuals from those of a calmer nature (Bryan, 1975). However, the definitions of panic in such research are usually vague and should cause us to view these data critically. Surely the nervous individual can be expected to treat danger cues in certain ways, but an acceptable specification of the link between personality and crisis is at present difficult to make.

Input 3: Current state factors

This is a somewhat difficult category, the components being included at times on the basis of operational as opposed to inherent set criteria. Essentially it comprises the sum of those variables external to the individual which describe his relationship to the environment and others present at the moment of cue detection (warnings, alarms, indirect cues, etc.).

(a)   *Component 1: subjective assessment of the environment.*
Once an individual senses that something is 'wrong' or unusual he is posed with the basic choice of continuing what he is doing or taking some form of action. The interpretation of the danger signal does not always seem to define whether action will or will not be taken. We have found in an analysis of a recent drill (unannounced) two people who did not take the alarm seriously. However, their reasons for taking action (leaving the building) were based on a type of economic trade-off argument. Both indicated that because the building was old, fire would spread quickly. Similarly they perceived themselves to be in a remote part of the building, which implied greater travel distance to an exit. They realised that an error in judgement resulting in no action would be worse where they were than, as one member of the Fire Research Unit was told, on the ground floor. The same error is therefore seen as having different consequences, depending on where one is.

(b)   *Component 2: perceived hazard exposure rate.* Building upon an index of fire risk used elsewhere (Crossman and Zachary, 1974), this component describes the occupants' perception of certain risks in the building, irrespective of location. If a person in an old structure knows that other tenants are using paraffin or wood fires, it is likely that cues and signals will be treated as indicating a real threat. Of course, the perception of hazard exposure rate and its objective value as determined by professionals need not coincide.

(c)   *Component 3: existence of expectancy cues.* These are attributes of the environment which, although we know little about them, can be thought of as potentially influential. A certain German university, for example, possesses a large lecture theatre with several break-glass units labelled 'Panic button'. Few have any idea of their function (emergency lighting) but new students sometimes attribute to the area non-existent dangers which could have some influence on behaviour. It might be possible to think of such attributes in terms of a self-fulfilling prophecy, that is, people could tend to behave according to the expectations they think others have of them.

In a similar manner, sign and notice wording may influence behaviour. The noted linguist Whorf (1956), while working as a fire inspector, was able to obtain evidence to this effect. He observed that 'gasoline drums' were treated with great caution, but, when empty, such caution disappeared. He interpreted this to imply that the term 'empty' predisposed those involved to interpret this as not dangerous. This was erroneous, given the potential danger from fumes.

(d)   *Component 4: Activity currently engaged in.* We found in the drill referred to above that people who were cooking dinner did not wish to evacuate. In fact, these were the only individuals to report being annoyed by the practice drill. It is conceivable that an alarm given while a group of conferees were having dinner would be greeted reluctantly if the fire risk were perceived as negligible. Wheeler (1968) speaks of 'inertial restraints' in such cases.

On numerous occasions the Fire Research Unit has noted a similar effect in those watching television. Quite often initial cues have been totally disregarded (including smoke drifting into the field of vision). This is not as peculiar as it might seem. Thus Stapelfeldt (1975) remarks, 'A student who saw the fire himself, first thought of his full glass which he emptied before going outside' (p. 10) or 'A girl called out "Fire!" to one of the musicians who thought he should play faster, as he himself reported later' (p. 10).

(e)   *Component 5: time of occurrence.* People have come to associate certain times of day or even of the year with regular rituals or events. Nearly all of those interviewed in a dormitory fire drill attended by the Unit took the alarm to be bogus because 'it was the beginning of term'. This time of year, it appears, is associated by the students with practice runs, thereby reducing the credibility of the signal. Cantril (1966) has reported similar 'timing' effects concerning a radio broadcast panic.

(f)   *Component 6: immediate role.* The role one exercises at the moment of receiving information (alarms, cues) appears to influence interpretation. Pauls (1971a) notes in one of his studies that members of staff who were also part of the Fire Emergency Organisation tended more than others to construe the event (alarm) as a real emergency. It is possible that the role sensitises. Alternatively, people in positions of responsibility for others (especially as this concerns life saving) do not wish to take chances and this attitude could permeate their private interpretations.

(g)   *Component 7: 'contrient' factors.* The name of this component has been taken from mathematical games theory and is used here to imply that the presence of another 'player' structures a game (cf. Deutsch 1949). The analogue to this in psychology is a 'yoked' relationship, that is, if you do something to one member of a relationship the action has related consequences for others in that situation. Something close to this occurs in many fire situations. We know, for example, that people with family members present will react to a crisis differently from others who are alone (Mack and Baker, 1961; Fritz, 1972). Moreover, a disproportionate number of people who re-enter burning buildings have family members inside (Wood, 1972). Many deaths in the Summerland resort fire were of this type and resulted from people searching for children (Report, undated). Abe's (1976) summary of behaviour during a nightclub fire points in a similar direction. In this case the link was between the manager and his clientele. In the Unit's studies of domestic fires the frequently significant role of neighbours has indicated a similar life-saving relationship. In effect, an appreciation of such factors will often indicate how inappropriate it may be to treat people in a crisis situation as independent or capable of pursuing the most effective actions. What some would construe as irrational or inadequate behaviour may be comprehensible once it is appreciated that, although some optimal path is perceived by the person, higher-order demands preclude advantage being taken of it.

This component can be seen to be closely associated with role (if not inseparable from it). One finds, in this respect, that alarms are taken more seriously by people immediately co-present with their families (Katz, 1960) or those with families removed from the immediate scene but within visiting distance (Mack and Baker, 1961).

Section Summary

As pertains to the recognition/interpretation stage, data obtained by the Fire Research Unit indicates unambiguously that the majority of people do not correctly interpret initial fire cues. Although the model as presented allowed for this possibility, the number of cases in which this has been found to occur has come as a surprise to us. Even in the case of what one might consider to be irrefutable and unmistakable indications of fire (the visible presence of smoke) people have invoked other explanations. We have found that the sound of smashing glass or people shouting and screaming becomes 'a fight outside', 'a party' or 'vandals'. People seldom associate odd noises with the possibility of a fire. Instead the noises are evaluated against a matrix of the familiar (Breaux, Canter and Sime, 1976).

In an attempt to dissect one fire situation for which we now have abundant data, the first run of a matrix analysis technique has even indicated that the early recognition and correct interpretation constitute a strong predictor of subsequent behaviour.

Indeed, given the focus in this volume on the domestic situation, it is worth noting that many of the costs involved in admitting that there is a fire in a person's home, such as social embarrassment or stopping ongoing pleasurable activities, are much greater than in a work setting, where officials anyway are likely to define the situation as a fire. Resultant reluctance to recognise early fire cues as such may be one of the reasons why domestic fires are so much more likely to be fatal than would be expected.

A further aspect of the domestic situation noted by the Fire Research Unit concerns the role on domestic routines. During the evening, dinner-time appears to be an overriding concept in the interpretation process during the early stages. In an attempt to account for why he took so long to react, an informant concluded 'I thought it was cooking anyway'. This raises an important point concerning the 'domestic' concept. One often tends to think of this in terms of a semi-detached or detached house in which one family or an extended version of it is resident. Many of the domestic fires investigated by the Fire Research Unit, however, have taken place in high-rise or multi-occupancy blocks. Apart from complicating the events with factors one may have attributed solely to non-domestic fires, incidents in such buildings further confuse cue interpretation. In the example cited above, neither the informant nor his wife was engaged in preparing dinner. In fact, upon smelling smoke, both thought that the family upstairs was cooking. In a similar incident three members of a family heard what they thought to be breaking glass in the early hours of the morning. This they attributed to 'partying' somewhere below them. From the above and other examples obtained by the Unit for such dwellings, it is apparent that the recipient of early fire cues need not personally be engaging in activities that would provide alternative explanations to the sensed stimuli. The presence of other families in the same building allows one to invoke normal explanations (to early cues) based on activities not personally engaged in. One expects an attenuation of the effect in detached or semi-detached homes. However, although there is a reduction in this class of explanation, its analogue occurs in that often it is supposed activities 'next door', 'down the street' or 'in the street' which form the basis of normalising causes.

Before concluding this section, a brief note concerning the role of television seems appropriate. On several occasions it has been found that although cues were perceived, investigation or attempts to explain them were postponed until a commercial or 'less gripping' part followed. This delay in dealing with the cues appears more pronounced for thriller and mystery programmes. Apart from a delay in dealing with them, such cues may also be totally overlooked. A similar phenomenon has been noted by one of the authors in parts of Germany and France for certain network mystery programmes. In this case numerous households were burgled while the victims were viewing the programme. Although several informants reported hearing strange noises, investigation was deferred until after the programme ended.

B. Stage II: Behaviour (action/no action)

After the evaluation process has been completed (or at some time concurrent with it) the information convinces the person that the situation is or is not dangerous. The possibility of taking action now arises. At the junction between Stages I and II four theoretical outcomes can be listed:

(1)   A person can accept the alarm or cue as indicating an emergency but take no action ('panic paralysis', remaining in the same place, etc.).

(2)   A person can construe the situation as a real emergency and take action (seek verification, leave, search, typical responses).

(3)   A person can assume the situation not to be an emergency but take action (perceived drill, 'playing it safe', social pressures to conform).

(4)   A person can assume the situation not to be an emergency and go about his normal routine.

Once action is taken (or even if no action is taken) there are several influential inputs (given the actual presence of a fire).

Input 1: Environmental factors

(a) *Component 1: impedance variables.* Smoke (Wood, 1972), heat, flames, travel distance, availability of exits, refuge areas, etc. — these clearly restrict the usual movement options available to an individual.

(b)   *Component 2: hazard factors.* Like the perceived hazard exposure rate above, this component can influence behaviour. If a person knows the fire to be near gas cylinders, rapid escape may occur with little other activity.

Input 2: Social factors

The effect of being with other people or the knowledge that one will eventually be in the presence of others. This latter point often seems to induce people to make themselves 'presentable' before taking action.

(a)   *Component 1: spacing demands.* Some groups might not evacuate as smoothly as planned due to the maintenance of body buffer zones even during an emergency (Pauls, 1971b). At times the maintenance of certain social conventions, even during times of crisis, may influence one's success in evading the danger (cf. LaPiere, 1938).

(b)   *Component 2: group characteristics.* Groups in which people know each other can be expected to behave differently from groups of strangers (Breaux, 1975; Westley, 1956). Similarly, it has been noted that groups in which a few children are seen to be present engage in less crushing (Westley, 1956).

Input 3: Salient components referred to under Stage I
(e.g. personality, role — designated by broken lines).

Section Summary:

In terms of the behaviour exhibited by those involved in fire situations, the Fire Research Unit has gathered information relating to action sequences. Whenever possible these data have been cross-checked with visits to the scene of the event and interviews with all those involved (including brigade personnel). An interesting and recurrent feature of fires which occur at night, especially in hotels, is that people will spend valuable time dressing and gathering belongings. Given that they have most probably ignored the initial cues, the fire by this time is likely to be characterised by non-linear growth. Thus every second spent on peripheral activity like dressing means a greater hazard to evade eventually. Further, the rate of growth often appears to increase in such a manner as to penalise severely those who waste time later in the sequence. Quite often, by the time an individual has correctly interpreted the cues and dressed, all means of escape except waiting by the window have become inaccessible.

At present the Fire Research Unit is investigating action strategies which seem to lead into behavioural cul-de-sacs. In the process it has been noted that certain patterns (e.g. entering a cycle of investigative behaviour only to end up by a window) appear to follow logically, given late recognition and dressing. Employing the same techniques (variations of matrix and linear analysis), an attempt is being made to offer a definition of the elusive 'effective behaviour' concept.

D. Stage III: Outcomes (evaluation and long-term effects)

At this stage the crisis is over and we can judge or evaluate the behaviour in restrospect. Depending on who does the evaluating, this stage can feed effects back into the system for future events. Thus design codes may be reinforced or modified on the basis of what is seen to occur over a range of incidents, or, at times, on the basis of one horrific event.

A second aspect of this stage concerns long-term effects on the individuals present during the emergency. Accordingly, the result of one's involvement might be to alter strategies of cue cultivation so as not to be caught unawares the next time (cf. Section A, 2(b)). Further, and of a more clinical nature, how has the fire affected people generally? Can we speak of traumas (Canter, 1975)? Studies (Zwingmann, 1971; Bonhoeffer, 1947; Panse, 1971) treating such factors in adults have failed to discern significantly detrimental long-term influence (excluding those who suffer severe injury, such as full-thickness burns and their attendant consequences.) However, the problem is complicated by definition of trauma, hospital treatment and labelling procedures, and the fact that those who do exhibit trauma often represent a self-selected population. It could be that people incapable of coping with a fire (either by containing or evading it) are psychologically different before the event.

(a)   *Component 1: psychological variables.* (personality, ability to cope with rapid environmental changes, ability to overcome shock and loss).

(b)   *Component 2: severity of loss.* (property and life).

(c)   *Component 3: publicity.* (the degree to which knowledge of the event reaches influential individuals or groups).

Section Summary

At present there appear to be few aspects of the situation as much in need of attention as the recognition/interpretation stage. From our research to date it is clear that a warning system is needed which will leave occupants in little doubt that there is in fact a fire. Additionally, such a system should be capable of communicating to occupants the size and location of the fire, thereby enhancing the likelihood that ineffective sequences are not initiated. All too often we have been able to trace an inability to escape unaided due to initial recognition delays. Cues must be made less ambiguous, although it is appreciated that this is not always an easy task. In part, research concerning tape recording systems is a move in this direction (Loftus and Keating, 1974).

Other long-term recommendations must await the accumulation of sufficient data. It is noted in passing that the project has already generated several spin-offs, one of these concerning how the public first contacts the brigade. Without going into detail, it is already apparent that techniques to facilitate the efficient transmission of information about, for example, the location of the fire, may be of great potential use to all concerned.

We are not as yet in a position to offer a critical examination of the long-term effects of fires on individuals. Moreover, the nature of such a question demands sufficient time to detect the effects if they exist. At present our main concern centres on an understanding of what people do in fires. We now know, at least, that the dynamics are of sufficient complexity to warrant further and detailed investigation on a number of fronts.

Notes

1. Unit width is a concept applying to the width of exits. It is based in Britain on the premise that the average width of an adult male at the shoulders is 530 mm (21 inches). Accordingly, two average people could move through an exit, side by side, if that exit were two unit widths across.
2. A *body buffer zone* arises from the tendency for an individual to maintain a space around his or her body, the penetration of which by others is undesired. This zone has been shown to vary depending on the people and situations involved. Other factors affect the area of the zone: for example, it tends to be greater in front of individuals than on either side of them.

References

Abe, K. (1976) The behaviour of survivors and victims in a Japanese nightclub fire: a descriptive research note. *Mass Emergencies* 1, 119-24.

Bonhoeffer, K. (1947) Psychopathologische Erfahrungen aus den beiden Welt-kriegen. *Nervenarzt* 18, 1.

Breaux, J. J. (1975) Factors Affecting Social Contagion in Crowds. Unpublished DPhil thesis, University of Oxford.

Breaux, J. J., Canter, D. and Sime, J. D. (1976) Psychological aspects of behaviour of people in fire situations. *Proceedings 5, Internationales Brandschutz-Seminar Karlsruhe*, vol. 2, pp. 39-50. Karlsruhe: V.F.D.B.

Bryan, J. L. (1975) Human behaviour in the fire situation. *Journal of Fire and Flammability* 6, 17-27.

Burch, D. (1971) Statement of Chairman Dean Burch, Federal Communications Commission. (Appearing before the Committee on Appropriations, House of Representatives, Washington, D. C. on 7 April 1971). Mimeo.

Canter, D. (1975). Psychological aspects of behaviour of people in fires. *Proceedings, Symposium on the Control of Smoke Movement in Building Fires*, vol. 1, pp. 59-67. Borehamwood: BRE Fire Research Station.

Canter, D. and Matthews, R. (1976) *Behaviour in Fires: The Possibilities for Research*, CP11/76. Borehamwood: BRE Fire Research Station.

Cantril, H. (1966) *The Invasion From Mars*. New York: Harper and Row (first published, 1940).

Crossman, E. and Zachary, W. B. (1974) Occupant response to domestic fire incidents. Berkeley: Dept. of Industrial Engineering and Operations Research, University of California. Mimeo.

Darley, J. and Latané, B. (1968) Bystander intervention in emergencies: diffusion of responsibility. *Journal of Personality and Social Psychology* 8, 377-83.

Deutsch, M. (1949) A theory of cooperation and competition. *Human Relations* 2, 129-52.

Evans, R. R. (1969) *Readings in Collective Behavior*, esp. Part 5. Chicago, Rand McNally.

Fritz, C. E. (1972) Comments on agenda for public response to hurricanes panel (Panel 4), Hurricane Preparedness Conference, Miami. Mimeo.

Globerson, S. and Crossman, E. (1972) Human factors in fire safety: literature survey and preliminary analysis. Dept. of Industrial Engineering and Operations Research: University of California. Mimeo.

Green, C. H. (1974) Measures of Safety. Unpublished Manuscript, University of Illinois.

Hansborough, T. A. (1961) *A Sociological Analysis of Man-Caused Forest Fires in Louisiana*. Louisiana State University.

Joyce, C. C. (1972) *The Status of Radio Warning Systems in the United States* (Defence Civil Preparedness, Note No. 264). Washington D.C.: US Government Printing Office.

Katz, E. (1960) Joy in Mudville: public reaction to the surprise sounding of Chicago's air raid sirens (working paper). Chicago: NORC. Mimeo.

LaPiere, R. (1938) *Collective Behavior*, New York: McGraw-Hill.

Loftus, E. F. and Keating, J. P. (1974) The psychology of emergency communications. Proceedings, Public Building Service International Conference on Firesafety in High-Rise Buildings. Mimeo.

Mack, R. W. and Baker, G. W. (1961) *The Occasion Instant: The Structure of Social Responses to Unanticipated Air Raid Warnings* (NRC, Publication 945). Washington D.C.: National Academy of Sciences.

Melinek, S. J. (1975) An analysis of evacuation times from buildings. *Proceedings Symposium on the Control of Smoke Movement in Building Fires*, vol. 1, pp. 50-8. Borehamwood: BRE Fire Research Station.

Murray, P. and Finch, P. (1975) Are you living or working in a death trap? *Time out* 262, 11-15.

Panse, F. (1971) Angst und Schreck, in *Katastrophenreaktionen* (ed. C. Zwingmann), pp. 3-17. Frankfurt: Akad. Verlagsgesellschaft.

Pauls, J. L. (1971a) Questionnaire Results for a High-Rise Office Building Evacuation Drill: General Purpose Building (confidential draft). Ottawa. Mimeo.

Pauls, J. L. (1971b) *Evacuation Drill Held in the B.C. Hydro Building 26 June 1969* (Building Research Note 80). Ottawa: National Research Council.

Pauls, J. L. (1974) Building evacuation and other fire-safety measures: some research results and their application to building design, operation, and regulation. Paper presented at the 5th Annual Conference, Environmental Design Research Association, University of Wisconsin. Mimeo.

Phillips, Anne W. (May-June 1975) The physiological and psychological effects of fire in high-rise buildings, *Factory Mutual System*, 8-11.

Quarantelli, E. (1973) Human behavior in disaster. Paper presented at Designing to Survive Disaster Conference, Chicago. Mimeo.

Report of the Summerland Fire Commission (undated) Isle of Man Government.

Slovic, P. (1972) Limitations of the mind of man: implications for decision making in the nuclear age, in *Risks vs. Benefit: Solution or Dream*, L.A. 4860 (ed. H. J. Otway). Springfield, Virginia: NTIS.

Stahl, F. I. (1975) Behavior based fire safety performance criteria for tall buildings. Paper presented at the 6th Annual Conference, Environmental Design Research Association, University of Kansas. Mimeo.

Stapelfeldt, J. P. (1975) Fire protection in dance bars and discotheques, Library

Translation 2063. Borehamwood: BRE Fire Research Station. Mimeo.

Turner, R. H. (1969) Collective behavior and conflict: new theoretical frameworks, in *Studies in Social Movements* (ed. B. McLaughlin). New York: Free Press.

Westley, W. A. (1956) *The Formation, Nature, and Control of Crowds* (DRB Contract HQ/Dev. 36), Canada: Directorate of Atomic Research, Defence Research Board.

Wheeler, L. (1968) Behavioral contagion: theory and research, in *Social Facilitation and Imitative Behavior* (eds. E. C. Simnel, R. A. Hoppel and G. A. Milton). Boston: Allyn and Bacon.

Whorf, B. L. (1956) The relation of habitual thought and behavior to language, in *Language, Thought and Reality: Selected Writings of Benjamin Lee Whorf* (ed. J. B. Carroll). Cambridge: MIT Press, and New York: Wiley.

Williams, H. B. (1964) Human factors warning-and-response systems, in *The Threat of Impending Disaster* (eds. G. H. Grosser, H. Wechsler and M. Greenblatt). Cambridge: MIT Press.

Wood, P. G. (1972) *The Behaviour of People in Fires* (Fire Research Note No. 953). Borehamwood: BRE Fire Research Station.

Zwingmann, C. (ed.) (1971) *Katastrophenreaktionen*. Frankfurt: Akad. Verlagsgesellschaft.

4 NATIONAL DATA FOR IMPROVING CONSUMER SAFETY

4a INTRODUCTION

Since October 1974 the responsibility for the safety of consumer products and home safety has been with the DPCP, the Department of Prices and Consumer Protection (previously, responsibility was with the Home Office). The objects of the consumer safety policy are set out in *Consumer Safety. A Consultative Document*, Cmnd. 6389 (1976), which states:

> The principal objectives of a consumer safety policy are to secure that:
> (i) goods available to the public present no undue risk to consumers;
> (ii) the public are warned about hazards which they may find in products and around the home and are advised on how to avoid them; and
> (iii) unsafe goods which are found on the market can be withdrawn from sale, or modified, quickly.
> In pursuing these objectives it must be remembered that higher product safety standards generally involve higher production costs which ultimately have to be paid for by the consumer. The benefits in each case have to be weighed carefully against the costs.

To meet these objectives, particularly the first, it is recognised that information is required about accidents and their causes. The three papers that follow relate to the research programme which has been set up, in part, to collect and evaluate such information. The research programme was started by the Scientific Advisory Branch of the Home Office, and since January 1976 has been the responsibility of the Safety Research Section attached to the Consumer Safety Unit of the DPCP. The factual details in the papers describe the Department's current work and plans for the future. Any views expressed are those of the individual authors and not necessarily those of the Department.

The first of these papers, 'The feasibility of Collecting Data about Home Accidents on a National Basis', describes a research project of between two and three years' duration carried out jointly by the Scientific Advisory Branch of the Home Office and the Institute of Consumer

Ergonomics. The second paper, 'Setting up a National System – Ideals and Reality', describes the current development work which will lead to a national data collection system. The third paper, 'A Framework for Home Accident Research and its Relation to Decision Making', describes the current research programmes of the Section. Particular emphasis is placed on the selection of areas for further research and the preventive actions to which the research has contributed.

4b THE FEASIBILITY OF COLLECTING DATA ABOUT HOME ACCIDENTS ON A NATIONAL BASIS[1]

C. Whittington

Current national data on home accidents refer only to those persons who are either admitted to hospital or die as a result of such an accident. Detailed information is restricted to the results of small *ad hoc* regional surveys, which, though valuable at a local level, cannot be considered representative of the national problem due to their typically small sample sizes.

The need for more reliable and up to date national information on domestic accidents is therefore clear. In view of this, a study was carried out by the Home Office[2] in conjunction with the Institute for Consumer Ergonomics, Loughborough, to assess to what extent such information could be obtained from existing sources. Organisation and planning of the study started in October 1972 and the majority of the data was collected during the period from July 1973 to June 1974.

The particular emphasis of the study was to attempt to identify domestic products or fixtures associated with home accidents,[3] with a view to defining priority groups of accidents which may require further investigation. The study was also intended to provide some initial estimate of the costs of accidents occurring in the home.

Agencies Involved in the Study

The agencies selected for inclusion in the study were hospital Accident and Emergency (AE) departments, General Practitioners (GPs), Health Visitors, Fire Brigades, Weights and Measures departments[4] and Coroners.

The reasons behind the choice of AE departments as the major source of data are self-evident. They provide access to sufficient data to allow various aspects of the problem to be examined; they have contact with a large number of accident victims, in the majority of cases fairly soon after the accident, and they have an existing administrative structure which already collects at least some information on accident cases. In order to obtain a realistic estimate of the size of the problem, the cooperation of GPs was also obtained. In addition, this provided some comparison between cases treated by them and those cases treated at AE departments. Health Visitors were chosen as the most appropriate group to carry out home visits to accident victims, since, although not professional interviewers, they are trained to observe the sorts of attitudes or circumstances which may be disadvantageous to the health and welfare of the family. Their work also brings them into contact with the range of individuals who have an increased probability of having an accident, i.e. the young and the elderly. In view of the orientation of the study towards consumer products, both Fire Brigades and Weights and Measures departments were approached for their cooperation, the former for information on domestic incidents attended by them and the latter for details of hazardous products which came to their attention.

Areas Involved in the Study

The choice of geographical area to be included in the study was based on a number of criteria.

(i) Defined catchment areas were required of a manageable size.
(ii) Each area had to be served by all the agencies selected to participate in the study.
(iii) For simplicity there had to be only one major AE department within each area.
(iv) The areas chosen had to reflect regional differences.

The six areas finally selected were the county boroughs (as defined by the pre-1974 boundaries) shown in Table 1.

Table 1   Areas Chosen to Participate in the Study

	Population (in thousands)
Huddersfield	131
Northampton	127
Norwich	122
Southampton	215
Gateshead	97
Bromley	301

Source: Registrar General's Statistical Review of England and Wales — Part II, Population Tables (1972).

The total defined catchment population within the six county boroughs was 993,000, approximately 2 per cent of the total population of

England and Wales.

Type of Information Collected by Each Agency

The types of incidents reported and the level of information collected by each agency are summarised in the following two tables. First, the medical services (see Table 2).

Table 2 Information Collected by the Medical Services

	Type of Incidents Reported	Level of Information Collected
Accident and Emergency depts	All cases of injury resulting from a home accident	The location of the accident and a brief description of the events leading up to it including any product involvement
Health Visitors	A sample of home accident cases identified at each hospital	Duplicate of hospital data for validation purposes plus some additional data
General Practitioners	All cases of injury resulting from a home accident	The location of the accident and a brief description of the events leading up to it

AE departments and GPs collected information on those home accidents identified and treated by them during the relevant study period. Health Visitors carried out follow-up visits to the homes of a sample of between 10 per cent and 15 per cent of those patients treated at the hospitals, both to collect additional and more specific information about the accidents and, by independently asking identical questions, to validate the information collected at the AE departments. They also obtained information directly relating to the economic impact of the accident on the individual or family.

Second, the remaining agencies (see Table 3). The Fire Brigades and Weights and Measures department were concerned mainly with identifying hazardous products and environmental features which came to their attention, independently of whether these were involved in any personal injury or property damage. Finally, coroners

Table 3 Information Collected by Remaining Agencies

		Type of Incidents Reported	Level of Information Collected
Fire Brigades	(i)	Fires in domestic premises	The location of the incident and a brief description of the events leading up to it including any product involvement and cost incurred.
	(ii)	False Alarms	
	(iii)	Special Services	
Weights & Measures dept		Hazardous products which come to their attention	The type and hazardous nature of the product

in each area reported cases of fatalities associated with home accidents which occurred during the study period.

The remainder of this paper will deal mainly with the involvement of the medical services, particularly the AE departments, since these reported the majority of cases and were concerned exclusively with incidents involving personal injury. Brief reference will however be made to the total number of cases reported by the remaining agencies.

Organisation of Data Collection in the AE Departments

The information collected within the AE departments was intended to provide a basis for selecting specific accident types and examining their underlying characteristics. However, because of pressures on both patients and clerical staff, only the most essential details of the accident location and the circumstances surrounding it were recorded. Emphasis was placed on the need to identify any products or environmental features involved in the accidents, and where possible a brief description of these was noted. The various categories of information collected within the AE departments are shown in Table 4.

The details shown in Table 4 were recorded on an appropriate A4 single-sided record sheet. In the main, this form was completed by hospital clerical staff, as they had initial contact with the patients as they arrived at the hospitals. There were two exceptions to this procedure. First, in Norwich, casualty doctors were involved in the collection of information. Second, in Southampton the existing casualty staff felt that they could not cope with the additional workload.

Table 4 Information Collected within AE Departments

PERSONAL IDENTIFICATION DATA	e.g. age, sex, data, etc.
STRUCTURED DESCRIPTIVE DATA	e.g. location, injury, etc.
UNSTRUCTURED DESCRIPTIVE DATA	details of circumstances leading up to the accident
PRODUCT DATA	details of products involved in the accident

A clerk was therefore employed by the Home Office to complete the forms required for the study. This clerk worked, as far as possible, the relevant hours to cover the peak periods for home accidents. In her absence the remaining clerical staff marked the Casualty Register to enable her to extract basic details for each case and also to follow up cases of possible re-attendance. Once all the available details were recorded, the completed forms were collected periodically and returned to the Medical Records Officer or a specially selected member of the casualty staff, who then returned them to the Home Office on a weekly basis.

Role of the Health Visitors in the Study

Each week a sample of cases was selected for which details were to be forwarded to the Health Visitors. This sample consisted of all in-patients who had been discharged within the previous week and 20 per cent (allowing for a degree of non-response) of the out-patients resident within each county borough. The details consisted of only personal data relating to the victim together with the date of attendance at hospital. Information relating to the circumstances surrounding the accident and to any product involvement was collected independently by the Health Visitor at the home of each patient. Prior warning of such a visit had been given at the hospital on a card distributed to all home accident victims.

Role of the General Practitioners in the Study

Evidence suggests that personal contact with the relevant doctors is needed to obtain successfully the cooperation of GPs in a study of this kind (Roberts and Payne, 1973). Only two of the areas were therefore chosen to be involved in this section of the study. This allowed the majority of the practices with patients resident in the county boroughs of Northampton and Gateshead to be visited personally by one of the members of the study team.

The doctors in these areas were asked to participate for the last three months of the overall study period of July 1973 to June 1974. A questionnaire was completed for all patients who were seen either by a doctor or a nurse as a result of a home accident. Patients who were referred either by telephone to the AE departments or who were sent directly from the surgery to the hospital, without being seen by either a doctor or a nurse, were not included in the survey. The information collected was kept to a minimum so that the workload on the doctor was of an acceptable level. No attempt was made to record any detailed information relating to products which may have been involved, since perusal of data already collected within the AE departments had indicated it would be feasible to extract sufficient product data from the unstructured accident description.

Since the completion of the study form required no assessment of a medical or diagnostic nature, it was left to the decision of the individual practices as to whom, either doctors or clerical staff, was made responsible for obtaining the information from the patient. Leaflets and posters were however provided for the waiting room, to encourage and motivate the public to report the accidents.

Overall Response

At the end of the study year a total of 16,675 reports had been obtained from the six agencies. These were distributed as shown in Table 5.

Table 5 Number of Cases Reported by each Agency

	No. of cases reported
AE departments	13,535
Fire Brigades	1,389
Health Visitors (sample of cases reported to AE departments)	1,107
Weights and Measures department	51
General Practitioners (2 areas/3 months)	561
Coroners	32
TOTAL	16,675

Before examining in detail the levels of response obtained in terms of either individual agencies or areas, the fundamental problems of classifying and establishing the reliability of the data will be discussed. Again only data collected by the medical services will be considered.

Classification of the Data

The major difficulty lay in coding the descriptive information relating to the type and cause of each accident, and the nature of the product involvement. In the coding framework devised, an attempt was made to retain the maximum information about the actual circumstances leading up to the accident. First, this unstructured information was used to produce four categories to describe the accident situation. A brief description of these four categories and the function each served is given in Table 6.

Due to the frequently complex ways in which products and household fixtures were associated with the accidents, the coding framework devised allowed for up to three products to be coded for each accident. In addition, it specified the way in which they were involved in the accident. This was done by posing a series of specific questions for each type of accident and coding the products in answer to these questions. An example of how this was done is given below.

Example of product coding

'A child playing upstairs, started to run downstairs, tripped over a toy and fell to the bottom of the stairs where he cut his hand on a chair'

Accident Type	:	Fall on stairs
Activity	:	Playing
Secondary Activity	:	Running downstairs
Action precipitating accident/injury	:	Tripping over object (toy)
Injury	:	Cut

Products/Features of house

Q.1.	What did the victim fall down/over?	:	Stairs
Q.1.	Did any product precipitate the fall?	:	Toy
Q.3.	What product did victim come in contact with during or after the fall?	:	Chair

---

Table 6 Coding Scheme for Unstructured Data

	Category	Description	Function
1. Accident Type	e.g. Poisoning Fall Inhalation Ingestion	Based on ICD* classification but expanded to provide a more realistic framework for coding minor accidents. One further sub-division was available if more detailed information was given.	This allowed comparison to be made between the results of the study and figures available for fatal accidents. Also, since the specific injury associated with the accident was recorded separately, this allowed the spectrum of injuries relating to particular types of accidents to be examined.
2. Major Activity	e.g. Household maintenance Food preparation	The major activity that the person was involved in when the accident occurred. Two further sub-divisions were available if more detailed information was given.	This indicated the activity or groups of activities which were associated with different types of accidents. Comparison with 'exposure' data from other studies could be used to isolate 'hazardous' activities.
3. Secondary Activity	e.g. Kneeling Standing Running	The physical or bodily movement the person was engaged in when the accident occurred.	Each major activity was frequently accompanied by a description of a physical or bodily movement in which the person was engaged. It was decided to extract this information to see if any of these groups of movement was associated with particular types of accidents or injuries.
4. Action precipitating the accident/injury.	e.g. Trapping part of body in/dropping/breaking/smashing.	The person's involvement in the accident and the events which led up to it.	The description of the accident varied as to what extent the person was involved in the events leading up to it. A tentative attempt was therefore made to classify this information so that the maximum amount of information about the accident could be retained.

* International Classification of Diseases.

Each product was represented by a four digit code. These codes were organised so that they could be accessed in two ways. First, within an alphabetical listing of the products and second, within overall major product groupings. Each individual accident description was coded independently by two coders, first on to a duplicate of the report coding section and then on to the report itself. These were then compared; when there was any disagreement between the two, a final decision was taken by an arbiter who then, when necessary, amended the coding on the original report.

Level of Information Available from the AE Departments

Bearing in mind the method of classification employed, the level of information on individual accidents available from the AE departments can now be examined. This is most easily done by considering the number and percentage of cases for which major variables had to be coded as 'unknown'. The variables can conveniently be split into two categories. First, those which are normally recorded at the AE department — age, sex, day of week of report and time of report. Second, those recorded specifically for the study — location of accident, accident type, activity, major injury type.

In the following two tables data from both Huddersfield and Southampton have been excluded. In Huddersfield consistent under-reporting was identified, whilst in Southampton the employment of a casualty clerk for only eight hours per day meant that only very brief details were recorded for the rest of the twenty-four hour period. This resulted in an abnormally high proportion of unknown data values. Table 7 refers to data normally recorded at the AE department. Overall, the number of cases for which this information was not available was minimal, in the region of 1 per cent.

Table 7 Data Normally Recorded at AE Department.
Number of Cases where the Value of a Variable was Coded as Unknown

Variable	Number of cases	Percentage of total cases reported
Age and sex	175	1.9
Day and week of report	0	0.0
Time of Report	96	1.0

Table 8 refers to data recorded specifically for the study. As expected, the highest completion rate was found for variables which were normally recorded by the AE departments. Nevertheless, with the exception of activity, information on the other variables was available for the large majority of accidents. The location of accident was however unknown in nearly 20 per cent of the cases.

Table 8 Data Recorded Specifically for the Study.
Number of Cases where the Value of a Variable was Coded as Unknown

Variable	Number of cases	Percentage of total cases reported
Location of accident	1,841	19.6
Accident type	497	5.3
Activity	4,668	49.6
Major injury type	713	7.6

Level of Product Information Available

As previously described, the coding framework devised for the products allowed for up to three products to be coded for each accident. This was done by posing a series of specific questions for each type of accident. Table 9 shows the number of times responses were obtained for the four major accident types identified.

Table 9 Level of Product Information Collected

Accident Type	Product Coded Position 1	Product Coded Position 2	Product Coded Position 3
Poisoning	897 (98.4)	59 (6.5)	58 (6.2)
Falls	3,292 (84.8)	577 (14.4)	410 (9.3)
Burns and Scalds	630 (93.2)	332 (49.1)	100 (14.8)
Cuts and Bruises	2,826 (78.9)	1,171 (39.7)	103 (4.1)

The product coding frame also allowed for additional information on the brand or age of the product to be noted. Dependent on product position, additional information was recorded in 10 to 16.4 per cent of the cases.

Reliability of the Data on Individual Accidents

The duplicate information collected by the Health Visitors was used to provide a check on the reliability of the data collected at the hospitals. The AE data and the Health Visitor data were matched record by record and the values of a number of variables compared. The variables chosen were accident type, location, occupation of victim and the activity of the victim at the time of the accident. The two sets of information were found to differ in three ways. First, the level of detail available about the accident; second, real disagreement in the detail available about the accident; and third, inconsistent use of the coding frame. The discrepancies found for each of the four variables compared will be briefly discussed in turn.

Accident type

Superficially there was disagreement in 41 per cent of all matched cases. However, in the large majority of these (83 per cent) the accident type was classified as unknown in one of the descriptions, usually in that recorded at the AE department. The main confusion was found in the Cuts or Bruises/Loss of Balance or Falls categories. In the main these confusions were due to minor differences in the accident description. For example, one description would say 'bumped head on coffee table' (which would be coded as a Cut/Bruise) and the other would say 'fell against coffee table and bumped head' (which would be coded as a fall).

Location

Again, there was superficial disagreement in 49 per cent of all matched cases. However, in 69 per cent of these the location was classified as unknown for one agency. Only 178 of the 1,047 cases showed real disagreement; the majority of these were understandable confusions, for example, between dining area and living room.

Occupation of victim

Only 13 per cent of all matched cases showed disagreement. The greatest confusion was experienced with the definition 'housewife', the 'employment' and 'referred' categories. This was largely due to lack of consistency with which this type of information was recorded at the hospital and also the failure of the coders to act systematically in classifying the data.

Activity

There was superficial disagreement in 47 per cent of all matched cases, though again 89 per cent of these were because the value of the variable was classified as 'unknown' in one of the descriptions. The only significant confusion was between the categories of Children Playing and Eating/Drinking. When these were investigated it was found that the accident description frequently included both descriptions — for example, child playing, swallowed button — and therefore there was no serious disagreement between the two sources of data. The major reason for any discrepancy was the ability of the Health Visitors to gather more extensive information in the home environment, thus minimising the number of times individual variables were classified as unknown.

Response Rates

Since they provided by far the largest source of data, individual response rates will be considered in detail for each of the AE departments involved. Table 10 shows the response rate within each area in terms of the estimated number of home accidents per 1,000 population per annum. It should be borne in mind that the catchment areas of each AE department are undefined but known to be larger than the respective county boroughs. Any calculation of rates (i.e. incidence per unit of population) involves using only those cases of persons resident within the old county boroughs. This means that a defined population base can be utilised.

It can be seen that the response rate ranged from 1.8 per 1,000 population in Huddersfield to 15.9 per 1,000 population in Norwich.

This wide variation in reporting rates is also illustrated in Table 11, which shows the home accidents reported as a percentage of the total new attendances for each hospital. This ranged from 0.8 per cent for Huddersfield to 11.6 per cent for Norwich.

When considering response, differences in reporting rates between areas may be attributed to a variety of causes.

(i)   Real differences may exist in the number and type of accidents occurring.
(ii)   Differences may reflect regional patterns in the usage of medical services.
(iii) Differences may be due to variation in the conscientiousness with which reports were completed or in the interpretation applied to the definition of home.

Table 10 Number of Home Accidents Reported per Unit of Population

Area	Population in County Borough* (in 1,000s)	Home Accidents occurring in and out of County Borough	Home Accidents occurring in County Borough	No. of Home Accidents per 1,000 population per annum
Bromley	301	897	746	2.48
Gateshead	97	4,691	1,516	15.6
Huddersfield	131	304	241	1.8
Northampton	127	1,701	1,036	8.2
Norwich	122	4,111	1,949	15.9
Southampton	215	3,831	2,533	11.8
Total	993	13,535	8,021	8.1

* *Source:* Registrar General's Statistical Review of England and Wales — Part II, Population Tables (1972).

Table 11 Number of Home Accidents Reported as a Percentage of Total New Attendances

Area	Home Accidents occurring in and out of County Borough	Total New Attendances (1973)*	No. of Home Accidents/ Total New Attendances
Bromley	897	29,335	3.1 %
Gateshead	4,691	31,194	8.6 %
Huddersfield	304	36,974	0.8 %
Northampton	1,701	38,838	4.4 %
Norwich	4,111	35,409	11.6 %
Southampton	3,831	38,173	10.0 %
Total	13,535	209,923	6.4 %

* *Source:* Department of Health and Social Security Statistics, 1973.

Unfortunately, due to the lack of any standard recording procedures on home accidents within the medical services, it is impossible to check accurately the extent to which under-reporting may have occurred. A number of checks were, however, possible in some of the areas.

The most thorough check was carried out in Gateshead, since an adequate description was consistently available in the Casualty Register to enable all the home accidents treated to be subsequently identified. It was found that the study results represented 100 per cent reporting of home accident cases; since comparable reporting rates also occurred in Norwich, it suggests that this area had also notified its full quota of domestic accidents. The reporting rate from Southampton was considered reliable due to the presence of the clerical assistant employed by the Home Office who had carried out a continuous check of the Casualty Register; however, many of the accidents were only briefly described. No checking procedure was possible in Northampton since home accidents were not routinely identified in hospital records.

In Bromley, it was suspected that a misunderstanding had occurred, since despite the request to report all home accidents, the clerical staff were tending only to report obvious 'product involved' injuries. At the completion of the study a check was made by inspecting a 10 per cent random sample of all the new attendances at Bromley. As a result it was estimated that the completed forms represented only some 25 per cent of the total number of home accident cases which were treated at the hospital during the study period. Finally, although repeated contact was made with the hospital to identify if any particular problems existed, obvious under-reporting occurred at Huddersfield. Since it was impossible to assess reliably the extent of this, the data from Huddersfield have not been included in the majority of analyses performed.

Comparison of Study Results with National Statistics on Home Accidents

Table 12 shows the relationship between the study results and national data available on deaths and hospital admissions due to home accidents. It can be seen that the ratio of the incidence of deaths to the incidence of hospital admissions and the total number of patients treated at AE departments is 1 : 19.6 : 163.2 for males and 1 : 15.5 : 111.0 for females. The study also revealed the important role played by the family doctor in the treatment of domestic accidents. The overall GP reporting rate was approximately two-thirds that of the AE departments. However, the large overlap in the treatment of cases must be emphasised. It was found that almost 33 per cent of the patients seen by the GPs had received previous hospital treatment. In addition, nearly 19 per cent of the cases seen initially by the GP required referral to hospital.

Table 12 Home Accidents: Comparative incidence of deaths, hospital
admissions, AE department cases and General Practitioner cases,
per million population per annum

	Male	Female
Deaths[1]	87	153
Hospital admissions[2]	1,702	2,380
Patients treated at AE departments[3]	14,200	16,990
General Practitioners[4]	9,020	10,500

Source:
1. Registrar General's Statistics, 1972.
2. Hospital In-patient Enquiry, 1972.
3. Feasibility Study, 1973-4, using results from Gateshead.
4. Feasibility Study, 1973-4, using results obtained in two study areas for a
   three-month period.

Discussion

In general it has been shown that the approach adopted in the feasibility study was an effective method of gathering information on home
accidents. The study reports were, in the main, well completed, and
although some under-reporting did occur, the overall level of response
was high, considering the relatively long study period, the lack of any
local organisation and the already high workload of the staff involved.

A number of limitations in the approach were however identified.
As anticipated, the AE department is not a suitable situation for
collecting detailed product data. In only a few cases was any further
information given on, for example, the brand or age of the product.
In many cases the patient may not know such details, or could give
misleading information. Neither can the data collected at the AE
department determine reliably the extent to which the product is
responsible for the occurrence of the accident. In-depth investigations
at the scene of the accident will invariably be needed to define the
complex interaction of person, product and environment within the
accident situation.

However, the results and recommendations emanating from
the study have provided the basis of the planning phase for the National
Surveillance System on home accidents currently under development
by the Department of Prices and Consumer Protection (DPCP, 1976)
and it is considered that such a monitoring system would provide a
valuable tool for establishing priorities for action and for evaluating
the effects of any preventive steps that are taken.

Notes

1. The work described in this paper was carried out by Louise Hesketh of the Home Office and Claire Whittington of the Institute for Consumer Ergonomics, Loughborough.
2. Prior to October 1974 the Home Office was responsible for the safety of many consumer goods and had power under the Consumer Protection Act (1961) to legislate on their safety aspects.
3. The definition of home used in the study was as follows: (i) house, apartment, or flat, garage and other domestic out-buildings of dwelling house; (ii) the area surrounding the house, such as a garden, yard, path, steps or driveway; (iii) institutions, such as homes for the elderly or student halls of residence; (iv) places of temporary accommodation, such as a caravan or houseboat.
4. Weights and Measures departments are now referred to as Trading Standards departments.

References

Department of Health and Social Security and Office of Population Censuses and Surveys (Annually) *Report on Hospital In-patient Enquiry, England and Wales* London: HMSO.

Department of Prices and Consumer Protection (1976) *Collection of Information on Accidents in the Home.* London: DPCP.

Office of Population Censuses and Surveys (Annually) *Registrar General's Statistical Review of England and Wales for the year . . .*, Parts I and II. London: HMSO.

Roberts, J. L. and Payne, V. (1973) Health and social costs of home accidents. Proceedings, RoSPA National Home Safety Conference. London: RoSPA. Mimeo.

4c SETTING UP A NATIONAL SYSTEM – IDEALS AND REALITY

R. Page

Introduction

As this is the second part of a three-part presentation, there will be few details, except where required to indicate continuity, on the results of the feasibility study or the proposed future development of this work. By this stage, too, the case for the introduction of such a national system should be fairly apparent. The objectives of this section of the accident surveillance system are to collect data from Accident and Emergency (AE) departments, which will: (i) provide reliable, comprehensive and nationally representative information; (ii) enable accidents which are amenable to action to be identified so that they can be investigated further; (iii) monitor the accident problem so that new hazards may be identified and new trends in known hazards investigated. This paper is basically a discussion of the extent to which these aims are likely to be modified by the constraints applied by the real world, and the techniques which are used to minimise these conditions.

Problems of Definition

The Department of Prices and Consumer Protections (DPCP) has responsibility for home safety. This embraces most home hazards, the main subjects excluded being fire prevention as such and safety aspects of the structure of the house. In addition, many accidents are interactive: for example, a person may fall down a flight of stairs and cut themselves on a pushchair which is stored at the bottom. Obviously the person collecting the data cannot ascertain the responsibility for the safety of the article involved at source, i.e. when the accident is reported at an AE department. Further, it may not be apparent at any stage: for example, where an accident is solely described as 'victim fell over'. Therefore, in practice, all accidents in the home (where these are strictly defined) must be included in the collection procedure. This completeness is in fact very necessary, as the whole range of articles involved in accidents needs to be seen in perspective. It is not sufficient to identify so many thousand accidents a year involving consumer products: one also needs to know how this figure relates to the total number of home accidents.

So, information will be collected about all accidents in and around the home, from which the DPCP and other departments and interested bodies may be able to obtain relevant statistics. From this we will then be able to carry out in-depth studies on areas of particular interest and provide other groups with background information on their areas of research.

Incorporation of the Recommendations of the Feasibility Study

In any developing scientific study, the results of a previous stage should be taken into consideration in succeeding stages. To this end it is useful to go through the recommendations of the feasibility study to show how the national system will attempt to cope with the shortcomings and anomalies identified by that study. The following points were noted:

(i)   The hospitals should be selected so as to be nationally representative. This has been done by the Office of Population Censuses and Surveys (OPCS) in their selection of the sample for the final stage. It covers the problem of calculating rates and avoids introducing complex weighting factors.

(ii)   A person should be employed by the DPCP in each hospital to supervise the data collection and to complete the coding. This has been done for the current development phase and has given us greater control over the data collection. This is consistent with experience in the USA where researchers are introducing more of their own staff at the data collection stage. In the national scheme the duties of the person involved will be fully specified. It is intended that we assist in their selection since we have found that the quality of the data depends to a great extent on the interest of the person employed in this position.

(iii)   A system of monitoring key variables from each hospital is needed to ensure that form completion rates are maintained at a high level. It is envisaged that this will mainly be carried out by our clerks, as they will be checking completed forms against all home accidents noted on the casualty register at the hospital desk. They will also be responsible for the maintenance of standards in the quality of the actual data. The introduction of regional coordinators should further these aims and help sustain an interest in the project.

(iv)   A more cost-effective method of validating the data should be considered. In the development phase, therefore, as well as for an interview validation method, two versions of a postal validation are

being tested. If either of these gives satisfactory results, they may
well be used for validation, and interviews will be used only for in-
depth studies. It should be noted that the patient's permission is
required for any follow-ups: in the development phase we are
obtaining an agreement rate of about 70 per cent (in many of the
remaining cases the victim had not been asked so actual refusals are
quite low).

(v)   The accessibility of the data was questioned: it was thought that
the accident description could be assessed via a microfilm retrieval
system or some other technique. It would be useful for the data
collection form to be microfilmed in any case because of space
considerations and security aspects. So, provided the volume of cases
to be assessed is fairly low, a simple retrieval system using a microfilm reader would be adequate. This would involve obtaining a
computer listing of cases required, looking up each case via a hospital
casualty number code and, where necessary, obtaining a hard copy
of the original. A further option currently being tested is for an
abbreviated (if necessary) version of the accident description to be
'coded' on to the computer, thus giving an automatic retrieval system.

(vi)   The possibility of including 'part of body injured' in the
information collected was mentioned. This is currently being tested
and likely to be included. It is hoped that this further detail of the
injury may give more accurate costings in further work on a priority
model to assess the relative expense of accidents in the home.

Hospital Procedures

The AE departments of which we have experience all have roughly
the same procedure as regards their paperwork. In most circumstances
the victim (usually accompanied) arrives at the reception desk where
personal details and brief details of the accident are entered on a
casualty card and into a casualty register. Each entry in this register
has a unique casualty number which is used as a reference point for all
documents related to the accident. In cases of severe injury, often
where the victim is brought in by ambulance, the person injured will
be seen by a doctor immediately and the receptionist has to obtain
details either from an accompanying person or the doctor, or from
the victim at a later stage. Fortunately there is in almost all cases an
insistence that every person entering the hospital for treatment must
appear in the casualty book. When the victim is treated, the casualty
card is completed by the medical staff, giving details of injury
and treatment and indicating whether he is admitted, discharged,

referred to a General Practitioner or any other procedure.

Obviously, our procedures have to fit in with those of the hospital. To this end the current data collection form is designed in two parts, the first incorporating information to be collected at the casualty desk, the second involving information obtained from the casualty card. Thus the receptionist is only involved in collecting part of the data, the rest being completed later by the clerk employed by the DPCP. Medical staff need not be involved at all, except where nursing staff act as casualty receptionists at nights. (Fuller details of the data collected are shown in Figure 1).

The actual procedures to be followed are shown in flowchart form in Figures 2 to 4 and are self-explanatory. The last of these is a set of administrative procedures required by the DPCP to code, validate and return the completed data collection forms. Again, these do not involve any current hospital staff. We have estimated that for eighty accidents a week the DPCP will require, at most, fifteen person-hours work a week at the hospital. The majority of this will be done by the clerical worker funded by the DPCP, except where he or she is not present at the reception desk (i.e. during the night) or when hospital procedures dictate that the data collection can be done by suitably trained existing staff. As we are considering twenty different hospitals, it will be appreciated that there has to be a degree of flexibility in this respect. The additional clerk is to be available for other duties when he or she is not working on the DPCP work. In any instance, the time taken on the accident surveillance scheme should be considerably less than the twenty-two hours per week a clerk is on duty, taking into account holidays, sickness, etc. (This figure was provided by an Area Health Authority Organisation and Maintenance section.)

For the national scheme the hospitals are approached by the Department of Health and Social Security through formal channels. The DPCP study team will then approach the hospital to set up initial contacts and to ascertain the most appropriate way of carrying out the data collection in the particular AE department. Then the contract staff, who are carrying out the day-to-day administration of the scheme, will follow this up by the interviewing of staff and subsequent training, introductions of forms and procedures, arranging for follow-ups, returning completed forms, and so on. This process serves to highlight the point that this national exercise cannot be seen as a 'one-off' survey; it has to be explicitly defined, unambiguous, and able to run smoothly with a minimum of intervention from DPCP staff.

Figure 1 Accident Information Collected

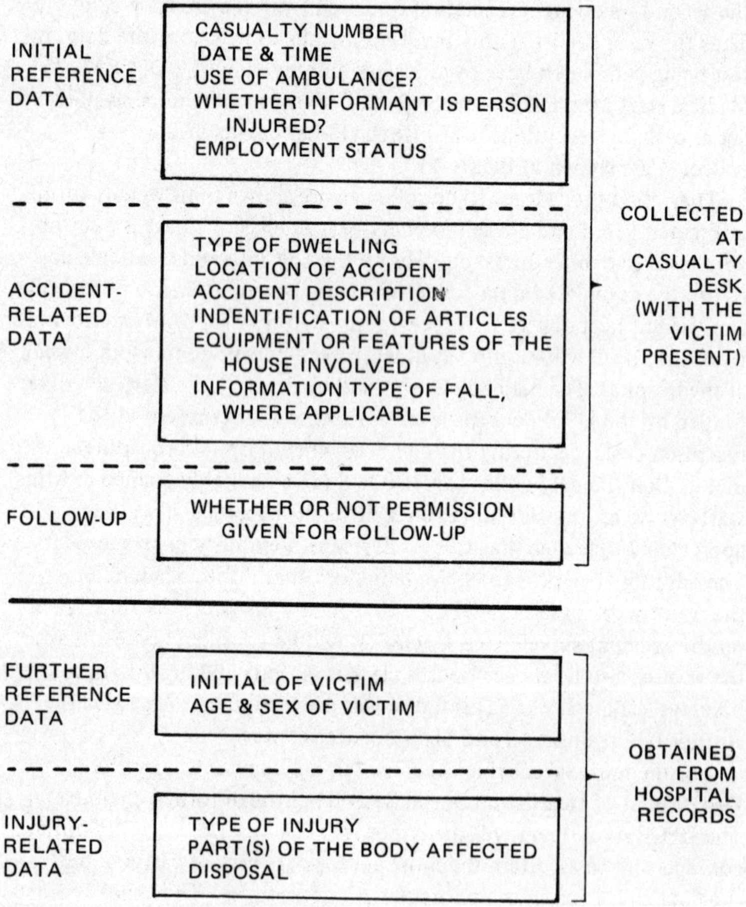

INITIAL REFERENCE DATA	CASUALTY NUMBER DATE & TIME USE OF AMBULANCE? WHETHER INFORMANT IS PERSON INJURED? EMPLOYMENT STATUS	COLLECTED AT CASUALTY DESK (WITH THE VICTIM PRESENT)
ACCIDENT-RELATED DATA	TYPE OF DWELLING LOCATION OF ACCIDENT ACCIDENT DESCRIPTION INDENTIFICATION OF ARTICLES EQUIPMENT OR FEATURES OF THE HOUSE INVOLVED INFORMATION TYPE OF FALL, WHERE APPLICABLE	
FOLLOW-UP	WHETHER OR NOT PERMISSION GIVEN FOR FOLLOW-UP	
FURTHER REFERENCE DATA	INITIAL OF VICTIM AGE & SEX OF VICTIM	OBTAINED FROM HOSPITAL RECORDS
INJURY-RELATED DATA	TYPE OF INJURY PART(S) OF THE BODY AFFECTED DISPOSAL	

Figure 2 Overall Data Collection Procedure

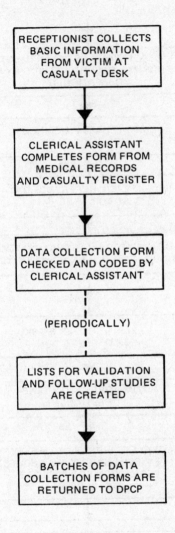

Figure 3 Completion of Details at Casualty Desk

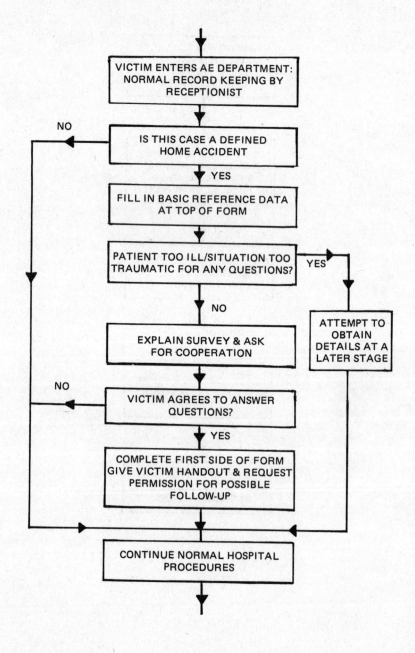

Figure 4 Periodic Procedures

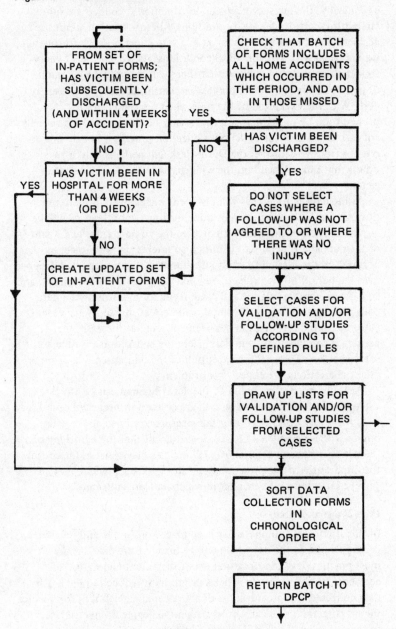

Practical Problems

Technically, the questionnaire and information it collects are quite
straightforward. Under ideal conditions, full information about the
accident could readily be obtained in a very short time. Unfortunately,
we are faced with far from ideal conditions. As we require a twenty-
four-hour coverage, it is likely that there will be quite a large number
of people involved in obtaining the basic information at the casualty
desk. With the exception of the time when our paid clerk is
present (and he or she may not necessarily be the person who actually
collects the data at the desk), the collection process is largely out of
our control. We can train the DPCP clerk and perhaps one or two
others, but must depend on the willingness of the casualty staff in
general.

As the national schemes will involve twenty hospitals scattered
throughout the country, two or three 'regional coordinators' will be
required. Their duties will be to oversee the completeness and quality
of the data and generally to maintain an interest in the project by the
hospital. In the feasibility study, the number of cases reported dropped
over the period of the project. We hope that the DPCP, by funding an
additional member of staff and more regularly monitoring the data
collection and visiting the hospital, will correct this to a large extent.
Once the initial information has been collected at the desk, the
process is completed by our clerk. Here the constraints on time are
somewhat less. So, with the exception of the odd miscoding or other
minor aberrations, we expect few problems.

Basically, then, the quality of the data obtained can be affected
where the staff at the casualty desk are either not interested or are very
busy (or both). It is hoped that the measures outlined above will
minimise these problems. In addition, it is felt that the launching of
the national stage in a more 'official' manner may assist in impressing
the importance of the project on casualty desk staff, which may in
turn be reflected in the manner in which data are collected.

Data Usage and Analysis

In this study great emphasis has been placed on simple and reliable
coding related to the use which will be made of the data. At the
most practical level, information about the extent and nature of
accidents involving certain articles or products will be required. The
data collected will provide a list of abbreviated case studies from which
the investigator will be able to ascertain the degree of involvement
of the article in question. Further, it will be possible to obtain

statistical tabulations of the data to isolate hazardous groups or locations of accidents or to compare the accident patterns of varying products.

On a wider scale, the production of statistics obtained from the data base is envisaged, including (as the sample has been chosen to be nationally representative) estimates of accident incidence over the whole country. It will also be possible for comparative statistics from, for example, one six-month period to the next, to be extracted. This could be required to monitor the extent to which new legislation is affecting the pattern of accidents in a particular field.

Looking further ahead, the data collected will be used as a base for on-going investigations and studies. In particular, the development of a priority model to highlight areas of high accident risk and cost will utilise data obtained from the surveillance scheme.

An Overview

From a scientific point of view, the accident surveillance system is quite straightforward. In the real world, which scientists sometimes find themselves having to work in, things are not so simple. To say that a single intractable casualty receptionist is going to alter national statistics is perhaps an overstatement; nevertheless, we shall have to monitor constantly the quality of the data collected. We have, however, had very good results from some of the hospitals currently involved in the development stage and, once a measure of goodwill is established in the hospitals in the national scheme, we feel confident of obtaining useful and reliable results.

Judging by the requests for information and interest shown following the publication of the feasibility study results, we feel that there is a demand for the information we shall be collecting. It has not been available in the past and so it is likely that we shall consider some sort of publicity, so that organisations who could make use of the statistics are aware that they are available. In any case, I am sure that most people will agree that it is a worthwhile exercise and goes a long way towards meeting the objectives of such a scheme.

References

Hesketh, L. J. and Whittington, C. (1974) Data Collection Feasibility Study on Home Accidents – Organisation and Implementation, Report No. 2/74, Part I. London: Home Office Scientific Advisory Branch, Accidents Study

Section. Mimeo.

Department of Prices and Consumer Protection (1976) *Collection of Information on Accidents in the Home.* London: DPCP.

4d A FRAMEWORK FOR HOME ACCIDENT RESEARCH AND ITS RELATION TO DECISION MAKING

C. A. Warne

Introduction

Broadly speaking, the Department of Prices and Consumer Protection (DPCP) has a responsibility to ensure that consumer products available to the public do not present an undue risk when in normal use. This paper does not consider the issues of 'undue risk' or 'normal risk', although the DPCP Safety Research section is well aware of these issues.

The ways in which the DPCP can execute this responsibility are outlined in the document on consumer safety, Command No. 6398 (DPCP, 1976b) published in February 1976. The Department acts in a variety of ways; direct actions include legislation (such as the Consumer Protection Act of 1961), and regulations about specific products (such as those referring to nightdresses), education and publicity, e.g. films for use on television. The Department can also devise, with relevant manufacturers or trade groups, codes of practice which are complied with voluntarily by the industry. The Department asks the British Standards Institute (BSI) to consider making standards relating to the safety of a product; and finally the Department handles a host of queries from individuals, local authorities and manufacturers about the safety of products. When considering the research programme the practicability of action in relation to a product or group of products is borne in mind. Such considerations have a definite influence on the framing and definition of the research carried out by or sponsored by the Safety Research section.

The role of the section is to carry out or sponsor research which will identify products or groups of products which are hazardous; allocate priorities for action between products; study in detail those products or groups of products found to be particularly hazardous; and evaluate the effects of different remedial measures in terms of accident reduction. This paper will consider the current activities of the Safety Research section in relation to this overall role and the actions available to the Department. The paper also aims to demonstrate, with examples, the way the current research has developed and the subsequent actions taken. Of course, one of the critical limiting factors is the resources available: currently the scientific staff consists of four members, one of whom works only part-time, very limited support staff, and a supporting extramural budget.

Surveillance Data

Some years ago now the relevant government department (then the Home Office) recognised that appropriate data were not available if the Department was to fulfil its obligations in relation to consumer safety in a systematic way. A limited programme of research was set up within a more far-reaching context. The most important project at that time was the feasibility study which aimed to look at existing data sources as a means of obtaining reliable information about product-related accidents at relatively low cost. This project and some of the results obtained have been discussed in the paper 'The Feasibility of Collecting Date about Home Accidents on a National Basis'. The information gained in this project has already been used to provide information on an *ad hoc* basis for BSI committees, various government departments and manufacturers, for consideration of priority for further research and to provide limited data to indicate the nature of hazards in relation to some products (DPCP, 1976a).

Two particular examples are:

(i)   Data from the feasibility study were used to establish which were the most common accidents associated with prams and push-chairs. The high incidence of falls from prams reinforced the case for specifying in regulations that adequate provision should be made for the mounting of safety harnesses.

(ii)   When the BSI standard relating to spin driers was amended, the statistics drew attention to the number of accidents involving spin driers. This reinforced the case for requiring that spin drier lids and doors should be so arranged that moving parts were not accessible whilst the container was revolving.

The successor to the feasibility study is the national surveillance system. This is currently in the final stages of development. Its aims and the types of issues currently under investigation have been considered in the paper 'Setting up a National System — Ideals and Reality'. Data collection on a national basis began at the end of 1976. Full analysis, of course, will not start until a reasonable amount of data has been collected. It is currently the intention that statistical information will be made readily available to all interested bodies and individuals.

The national surveillance system involves collecting and analysing data about those accidents in the home which are reported to AE departments and is the basis of the research programme of the Safety Research section. The system will provide some basic data about whether or not a hazard may exist in relation to a product. Such overall national data are not intended to define the actual hazards which exist in relation to a specific product. Specific in-depth research in relation to a product or group of products will normally provide detailed information about the way the products are involved in accidents.

Factors Affecting Priority for Study

The national surveillance system is therefore the first stage in identifying possible problem areas accurately, at least in terms of accident frequency. As all the possible problems identified cannot be studied at once, a method is required for allocating priorities in a systematic manner. Table 1 lists two sets of factors relevant to the selection of a product for more detailed study. The first group are factors about which objective measures can be obtained; the second comprises additional factors or issues which also affect the decision.

Table 1 Factors Affecting Priority

Objective Factors	Other Factors
1. Frequency	1. Amenability to solution
2. Severity	2. Cost-effectiveness
3. Cost — Medical Lost earnings, etc.	3. Accident or victim types
4. Risk	4. BSI and EEC interest
5. Product life	5. Political pressure
	6. Public pressure

Sadly, at any juncture, information is not necessarily available about all the objective factors. In practice, therefore, decisions have to be made in the light of the information available at the time. This was the situation when the first group of products, household products, was selected for in-depth investigation.

Selection of a Group of Products and their In-Depth Study

We will now consider briefly the in-depth study of household products[1] carried out for the Safety Research section by the Institute of Consumer Ergonomics (ICE) (Whittington and Wilson, 1976). Those aspects pertinent to the theme of this paper will be considered, but other aspects, such as the method, will be greatly condensed. It is expected that more information about the study will eventually be published. Those aspects considered include the rationale for studying suspected poisonings attributable to household products; some overall results which are pertinent to the remedial action that can be taken; and action in hand to study specific aspects of the problem further and to reduce the occurrence of these accidents.

Soon after preliminary results of the feasibility study became available, it was decided to select a product or group of products for more detailed study. In view of the small data base, i.e. cases from six AE departments only, it seemed realistic to select a group of products rather than an individual product for study. Similarly, it seemed realistic to select a group of accidents which appeared relatively homogeneous on the basis of the available data. This would increase the chances of obtaining reliable results from a small initial data base.

The accident types in relation to many products are very varied (e.g. bottles, which may be involved in cuts, falls and poisonings) and a large sample of accidents would be required for detailed study of any such product. There are some forty-five major groups of products in the analysis but only six broad accident types; it was useful to look in the first instance at accident type. A tabulation (see Table 2) of accident type by age showed that suspected poisonings were almost entirely restricted to children and that there were some 923 of these, representing about 9 per cent of the accidents identified in the feasibility study. None of the other major accident types looked so homogeneous. A tabulation of product against accident type also showed that two major groups of products were involved in these suspected poisonings — pharmaceutical and household products — and that about a third of the suspected poisonings were attributable to household products. A tabulation of injury type by severity (measured in terms of degree of treatment required) showed that 31.5 per cent of the suspected poisonings resulted in the patient being admitted to hospital. This was a higher percentage than for any other of the broad accident types (see Table 3). There were therefore good objective reasons for studying these accidents in depth.

Other important considerations which influenced the decision to

Table 2 Accident type analysed by age (AE Dept. Data: N = 13, 131) *

Accident Type	0-4	5-15	15-44	45-64	65+	Total
Suspected poisonings	793	122	8	0	0	923
Loss of balance, falls	1,218	670	909	632	947	4,376
Burns and scalds	248	102	180	85	33	648
Cuts, bruises, puncture wounds	625	638	1,412	527	230	3,432
Inhalation/Ingestion	73	12	16	12	5	118
Foreign body in orifice	51	26	39	15	4	135
Other specified	6	4	23	9	3	45
						9,577

* Cases in which the accident type was not specified have been omitted.

Table 3 Injury Tupe Analysed by Severity (AE Dept. Data: N = 13, 131)*

Injury Type	Out-Patient Only	Further Treatment	In-Patient	Fatal	Total
Suspected Poisoning	399 51.9%	132 16.7%	245 31.5%	1 0.1%	777 100%
Cuts/Bruises	3,548 68.4%	1,533 29.3%	128 2.5%	7 0.1%	5,216 100%
Dislocation/ Fracture	571 36.6%	581 37.3%	283 18.2%	23 1.5%	1,458 100%
Burns/Scalds	337 51.8%	246 37.8%	65 10%	3 0.5%	651 100%
Other	326 68.1%	68 14.2%	81 16.9%	4 0.8%	479 100%
Total	5,181 60.3%	2,560 29.8%	802 9.3%	38 0.4%	8,581 100%

* Cases in which the injury type was not specified have been omitted.

study suspected poisonings from household products were that first, it was widely held that the use of childproof closures and lockable storage would to a great extent solve the problem; second, the BSI were at that time developing a standard for childproof closures for pharmaceutical products: if a good case could be made, it was possible that this standard could be extended; and third, the European Economic Community (EEC) was interested in this problem.

The study used cases identified in the feasibility study and the further cases reported to those AE departments in the following eight-month period. Some 550 cases were identified and detailed follow-up interviews successfully carried out on 401, giving a response rate of 72 per cent. The most common reason for lack of response was change of address. Health Visitors carried out the follow-up interviews, using a detailed questionnaire designed by the ICE team after appropriate pilot interviews.

From the point of view of practical remedial action the following are some of the important findings.

(i)   Approximately 100 different substances were involved in the poisonings. Turpentine and turpentine substitute formed the largest single category, accounting for 67 (12 per cent) of the cases.

(ii)   The 6 most frequently named products (turpentine and turpentine substitute, bleach, paraffin, disinfectant, perfume and nail polish remover) accounted for about 40 per cent of the total number of cases.

(iii) With the exception of a small number of cases involving powdered bleach and some insecticides and rodenticides, all the substances with an absolute frequency of 10 or more were liquids.

(iv)   Of the products involved, 52 per cent were out of their normal place of storage when the accident happened.

(v)   Some 15 per cent had been removed from their original container. Among these cases, turpentine and other brush cleaners featured frequently.

A number of possible remedial areas were suggested. These included the provision and promotion of 'safe' storage in the home and modification of the product. Specific suggestions include the development and introduction of child-resistant closures for household product containers, the development of containers appropriate for the method of use of specific products, and a study of how people discriminate between containers. The need for research into aspects of labelling was also stressed.

Action has already been taken:

(i)   A case has been made to the BSI to produce a standard for child-proof closures for household products.

(ii)   Research has been commissioned to investigate in-depth solutions to the problem of products, such as turpentine and turpentine substitute, which by the nature of their use are transferred from the original container.

(iii)   Research has been commissioned to investigate and develop a series of symbolic hazard labelling for consumer products with special reference to household products.

Considerations of Length of Incapacity and Cost

As part of the feasibility study, Health Visitors were involved as one possible source of data about home accidents. They interviewed in the home about 13 per cent of the patients who had attended AE departments. It was possible in the atmosphere of the home to collect more detailed information than was collected at the AE department. Additional information that was collected included information about the length of the incapacity resulting from the injury. Length of incapacity was defined as the number of days off work or away from school, college, etc., or, for those not working, the number of days that the victim was unable to fulfil his normal duties. The mean number of days of incapacity for each of the broad accident types that analysis of the data produced is shown in Table 4.

A number of interesting points emerge. Dislocations and fractures, not surprisingly, result in long periods of incapacity. These accidents are mainly falls and many involve features of the house, e.g. stairs, rather than products. As such, they are not accidents which would be selected for study by the Safety Research section at this stage, as they fall outside the DPCP's responsibilities. The Department of the Environment is involved in research into accidents associated with stairs and, to a lesser extent, doors and windows. Burns and scalds as a class of accident type also involve very long periods of incapacity. Suspected poisonings, however, result in very low periods of incapacity.

The Health Visitors also asked about the time taken off work by people other than the victim as a result of the accident. The data in Table 5 show that in a relatively small number, 9 per cent of cases, a person other than the victim took time off work because of the accident to the victim. The average length of time taken from work

Table 4 Time of Incapacity (Mean Number of Days) (Health Visitor Data: N = 1047)

Injury Type	No Injury	Out-Patient Only	Further Treatment	In-Patient
Cuts/Bruises	0	7.7	15.8	17.3
Burns/Scalds	0	9.0	9.0	31.4
Dislocation/Fractures	0	20.3	38.3	53.9
Poisoning/Ingestion	0	1.0	1.0	1.8
Other	0	9.7	11.8	7.7

Table 5 Age of Victim Analysed by Accident Requiring Another Person to be Off Work (Health Visitor Data: N = 1047)

	0-4	5-14	15-44	45-64	65+	Total
Other person off work	32	16	19	14	13	94
	9.4%	9.4%	7.4%	9.7%	9.9%	9.0%
Total No. Accidents	342	170	256	143	131	1,042
	100%	100%	100%	100%	100%	100%

Table 6 Cost of the Medical Care (Mean Cost in Pounds, using 1973 Costs)

Injury Type	No Injury	Out-Patient Only	Further Treatment	In-Patient
Cuts/Bruises	9.91	10.83	11.72	80.49
Burns/Scalds	9.91	11.56	13.32	233.48
Dislocation/Fractures	9.91	15.20	19.78	366.99
Poisoning/Ingestion	9.91	9.91	9.91	26.20
Other	9.91	11.48	15.13	118.24

was 2.8 days, which is very small compared with the time of incapacity for the victim (see Table 4).

There are numerous ways in which costs can be attributed to accidents. There are two major aspects contributing to the cost of an accident: the cost of the medical care used and the loss of earnings, projected earnings, life years or equivalent. Considering the cost of the medical care, and using 1973 values,[2] the costs shown in Table 6 are produced.

Some preliminary calculations on lost earnings show that these are, overall, small compared with the medical costs. This is because the majority of home accidents happen to people who are not earning. It is not the subject of this paper to discuss the methods of costing home accidents and the implications of using different methods. John Roberts*(1973) has demonstrated the effect of the method used for costing on the allocation of priority among age groups. The only consistent feature to emerge was the importance of children and the elderly!

For the present, only the costs of the medical care involved are being considered. It has been shown that burns and scalds accidents result in both high medical costs and long periods of incapacity (Tables 4 and 6). Over half of these accidents also occur to children under the age of fifteen. During this year, therefore, we are examining aspects of this problem more closely. A study is being carried out by the Institute of Consumer Ergonomics of accidents in the kitchen with special reference to cooking accidents. The Safety Research section is setting up a study of accidents resulting in serious burns or scalds.

Risk of Injury

Of the objective factors which affect the allocation of priority to different problem areas, some information is already available about frequency, severity and cost. The aspect of risk is an almost untouched area. In the case of household products, a study of exposure to risk was carried out in parallel with and in the same geographical areas as the investigation of suspected poisonings. The study on exposure to risk considered eight products (turpentine, bleach, washing-up liquid, window cleaner, metal polish, surgical spirit, disinfectant and paraffin) in a sample of households which contained children under five. The results of the study do not alter the conclusions of the investigation of suspected poisonings but qualify some of the findings both in terms of demographic variables and features of the use and storage of the products.

The Safety Research section plans to consider the problem of exposure to risk in the present research programme. It is expected that considerations of risk will be particularly important in attaching due weight to products infrequently involved in accidents, e.g. sun lamps or spades.

Summary

This paper has attempted to illustrate the way that the basic data from a surveillance system is fundamental for a research programme into product safety. The national surveillance system collects basic data about product-involved accidents as economically as is consistent with the data being valid and reliable.

This basic data can be used as a keystone for an objective system of allocating priorities to studies of different hazardous products. The resulting possible high-priority areas for further action are then considered in the light of the other factors listed in Table 1. An in-depth study, usually involving follow-up of cases identified in the surveillance system, is then set up to tackle the selected priority area. Such studies aim to discover in detail what aspects of the product, features of its use, and characteristics of the user contribute to the hazardous nature of the product. In all cases the in-depth studies will be set up with a view to identifying possible preventive measures. It is fully expected that further investigation will be required into preventive measures, e.g. the current research in the household products area is concerned with studying in more detail the use of turpentine, turpentine substitute and some other products in which transference from the original container is inherent in their current method of use. In the longer term it is hoped that it will be possible to develop a model to evaluate different strategies of protective action.

Notes

1. Household products are expendable products used in and around the home which are not intended to be consumed. They do not include pharmaceutical products. They include cleaning materials, paints, garden chemicals, and, for the purposes of this study, cosmetics.
2. Average costs of medical care (1973 prices)

1 AE visit (new out-patient)	£ 9.9
1 day in-patient	£13.1
1 GP consultation (estimate)	£ 1.6

References

Department of Prices and Consumer Protection (1976a). *Collection of Information on Accidents in the Home.* London: DPCP.

Department of Prices and Consumer Protection (1976b). *Consumer Safety. A Consultative Document.* Cmnd. 6398. London: HMSO.

Roberts, J. L. (1973). Economics of home accidents — problems of assessing priorities for investment in health education programmes. Paper presented to the Health Economists Study Group. Bristol: Health Education Council. Mimeo.

Whittington, C. and Wilson, J. R. (1976). In-Depth Investigation of Suspected Poisoning in the Home Involving Household Products. Unpublished report. Institute of Consumer Ergonomics Ltd, University of Loughborough.

5 A CRITICAL REVIEW OF THE 1976 GOVERNMENT CONSULTATIVE DOCUMENT ON CONSUMER SAFETY

J. L. Roberts and J. W. Dale

Introduction

Since the Second World War there has been a growing interest in the problem of domestic accidents and what now comes under the more general title of 'consumer safety'. The need to create a safer environment for people has become an increasing priority as accidents take a greater proportionate toll of the young and middle-aged in all developed societies in which infective and parasitic diseases have been largely conquered. In the United Kingdom, 7,000 people die each year from domestic accidents and many others are killed in sporting, leisure and institutional accidents. These numbers now are not far short of the total accidental deaths in all road, rail and other transport accidents, plus industrial accidents in the United Kingdom. But they have received little attention from scientific researchers or public service investigators by comparison with other classes of fatal accidents. Accidents in industry are covered by the factory inspectors, those in the air are covered by air crash investigation teams, those involving railways are considered by the railway inspectorate, and accidents on the roads are covered by police and special investigation units of the Road Research Laboratory or by university departments, such as the Department of Transportation and Environmental Planning in Birmingham.

These investigation units have established systems and methods of undertaking detailed field work, laboratory simulation and other experimental studies, and to a significant although limited extent, field trials, to test prototype improvements in design of equipment, environmental features, operating procedures, and to develop training and education of technical and other staff and of the general public. These developments have largely passed by the problem of domestic accidents, which have remained for many years an almost uncharted field of enquiry. The result has been that the approaches to establishing priorities for action on home safety have remained essentially pre-scientific, more influenced by speculation and the buoyant fads and fashions of safety groups than related to hard facts of how accidents happen. Moreover, compared with the extensive legislation on transport and industrial safety, the production of home and consumer products has been left virtually free of control, open to anyone producing any product or environmental feature. Try any shoe shop and ask for a pair of safe slippers for granny. You can get pink, or white; but safe? No − the concept is not known.

For these reasons the consultative document published by the United Kingdom Department of Prices and Consumer Protection (DPCP) in February 1976 is welcomed (DPCP, 1976a; DPCP, 1976b). In this paper we examine some of the issues it raises, and some of the proposals it makes. We consider how far these proposals are relevant to what is known about the problems of consumer protection and accidents, from the limited evidence so far established. We consider how far the proposals are likely to cover the main gaps in that evidence and how far they will direct research and development to the key problems. Finally we set out what fresh proposals we consider are necessary to increase the likelihood that consumers will be safer henceforth.

Problems of Definition

The document, in the foreword, limits its attention to 'ways of reducing the cost and suffering caused by home accidents' and 'how the law can best ensure that goods which reach consumers are as safe to use as the public may reasonably expect'. It is not entirely clear how far the document and the proposed laws embrace the consumer in all his personal activities or whether they are strictly limited to his activities in the confines of his home and garden. Nor is it clear whether 'home accidents' include those activities frequently involved in accidents at home which do not simply involve movable consumer goods but are also related to more general design and architectural features or the peculiar interaction and unexpected combination of architectural design, movable consumer products, servicing arrangements and human behaviour. Two examples are that carbon monoxide poisoning resulting from the overgassing of open flue and unflued gas water heaters may not be covered by the Department's proposals,[1] nor falls on stairways precipitated by deficiencies in lighting, carpeting, footwear or maintenance. Both are examples of circumstances giving rise to large numbers of fatal and non-fatal accidents at home where the proposed systems and legislation may not give investigators an unlimited brief to study the causes and develop and implement remedies. But we shall return to these issues

later, as they raise more fundamental problems of research development
and control strategy than those merely of definition indicated here.

The Responsibilities of Other Departments

Home accidents are not entirely the responsibility of the DPCP.
Because of the historical organisation of responsibilities of government
departments, certain specific safety problems are out of bounds to the
DPCP. Some of these are of relatively minor importance in terms of
the total problem of premature death and injury — like fireworks and
medicinal products; others are certainly more pervasive factors which
need to be explored if only to screen out their influence from a very
large number of cases, for example drink (particularly alcohol) and
food. Other excluded topics of more importance, such as fire and
safety aspects of the structure of the house, are excluded from DPCP
responsibility. Fires which result in a call on the fire brigades are
investigated by Fire Prevention Officers and important research is
conducted by the Fire Research Station, but certain aspects of the
design of equipment involved directly in fires and in the results of fire
may be more productively explored under the aegis of new legislation
than by traditional methods: for example, aspects of the design of
cookers, heating equipment, the lay-out of kitchens, methods of
cooking, and procedures in installing, servicing and maintaining equipment, and the identification, purchasing and retailing of oil heaters and
the fuel for these — all these matters may be related to the safety of
the consumer from the risk of fire. We need to ask whether the present
responsibilities of the Home Office for fire prevention and those
undertaken by the Fire Research Station adequately cover these aspects
of safety from fire. We hope that the proposed legislation following
the consultative document will cover any such gaps in the system.

Cutting the Cost of Accidents

The consultative document states (p. 1) that the three main aims of a
consumer safety policy are to secure that: (i) goods available to the
public present no undue risk to consumers; (ii) the public are warned
about hazards which they may find in products in and around the home
and are advised how to avoid them; and (iii) unsafe goods which are
found on the market can be withdrawn from sale, or modified, quickly.
But better product safety may not be the best way of cutting the cost
of accidents. Product safety is a much more limited field of enquiry
than accident control. The foreword to the consultative document
is concerned with 'ways of reducing the cost and suffering caused by

home accidents', which suggests that it is concerned with domestic accidents, not just home safety or product safety. If we begin with the aim: 'to secure that the cost and suffering caused by home accidents is reduced', as the foreword begins, then a greater range of hypotheses are open to the investigator in pursuing the causes and remedies of accidents, compared with the limited pathway explored in the rest of the document. The approach of this document implies that particular controls on consumer products are a key to reducing the cost and suffering of home accidents.

We believe there are serious shortcomings in pre-empting the field of enquiry by setting out these proposals for a complex system of information collection about consumer products and the introduction of legislation to control them.[2] As a result, other important safety strategies may be ignored and other government departments and agencies with responsibilities for home safety may erroneously presume that the proposed safety system is all-embracing when it is not. The Department of Health and Social Security, for example, is remarkably silent about home accidents and may think the responsibilities of the DPCP cover all aspects of the problem.

The cost and suffering resulting from home accidents is measured in terms of premature death, the extent of human tissue damage, time off work, days of restricted activity, property damage and so on. It may be possible to reduce the cost and suffering of accidents more quickly and efficiently by improving systems of treatment of injury, by improving the organisation and performance of rescue services and of repair services, by better rehabilitation services, by more training of professional staff and more education of the general public in how to deal with accidents when they occur.

We may make a major contribution by house repairs or by repairs, maintenance, and modification to existing equipment in the home, to make the existing environment and the existing equipment safer, rather than by monitoring intensively the safety of new equipment and of new houses. The practices of the repair and maintenance industries therefore become a major topic for study.

The choice of seat belts as a major part of the control of road accidents, deaths and injury is a case in point. Seat belts are not a means of avoiding accidents but of reducing the injury. The design of rescue equipment, flares and first aid boxes to cope with sporting accidents is not to prevent accidents but to deal efficiently with their consequences. Improvements in first aid at home, the establishment of the optimum methods of medical and nursing care for injuries, the

evaluation of pathology investigations in establishing causes of
accidents, evaluation of physiotherapy related to traumatic injury and
studies of the 'industrial' rehabilitation of the housewife following
accidental injury, including field trials of prosthetic and other aids —
all these may have a greater impact on the problem and may be more
cost effective than the limited strategies implied in the document.
Certainly assurances are needed that first, proposed investigations by
the DPCP into the nature of the accident problem and its possible
remedies will not prohibit or create obstacles to the exploration by
other agencies and departments of alternative strategies to those to
which the DPCP may be limited. If the DPCP have a monopoly of
research and development funds on domestic accidents, only a small
part of the field of enquiry can be examined. Second, other agencies
such as the Department of Health and Social Security, the Department
of the Environment, and the Department of Sport should be positively
enjoined in the programme of study and control to ensure that the
ultimate objective of cutting the cost of accidents is pursued
comprehensively and not on too narrow a front.

The Bristol Project

We shall now examine these general points in the light of evidence
from the Bristol studies to which the consultative document refers
(p. 3, para. 10) and in which a small number of us were intimately
involved. The Bristol Project was conducted over a period of five years
from 1969-74 by the former Medical Research Division of the Health
Education Council.[3] It was a community-based project which covered
all the domestic accidents in a population of 127,000 people living in
certain defined, contiguous electoral wards in north east Bristol
(Roberts, Payne, Dale, Northover, Simmons and de Fonseka, 1974;
Dale, Roberts, de Fonseka, Simpson, Knight and Payne, 1974). A
positive search was made of all hospitals', general practitioners', fire
services' and coroners' records during a period of more than two years;
4,600 accident cases were investigated on site by at least one
investigator, and within this total about 10 per cent were investigated
in depth by experts within the research group or others called in or
associated with the project; for example, we subjected the following
groups of accidents to detailed investigations and have published
separate papers or research reports on most of them (Simpson *et al.*,
1974; Gill, 1973; Lord, 1974; Yeats, Roberts and Dale, 1974; Slater,
1973).

1. cases of suspected and proven child poisoning
2. falls from ladders and steps
3. falls on stairways
4. cases involving architectural glass
5. carbon monoxide poisoning from gas water heaters
6. scalds from kettles
7. chip pan fires
8. cases involving food tins
9. fatal accidents
10. locations and particular streets with a high incidence of accidents within the study area.

It is disturbing to note how few of these topics which we considered the best for special study are directly within the limits of the proposed legislation and the proposed investigation system set out in the DPCP document.

Associated with the main research were other special investigations. These included: (i) the incidence of injury not resulting in use of health treatment or fire services; and (ii) legal aspects of accidental injury and fire damage in the home.

Following the unexpected closure of the Division by the Health Education Council, much of the material remains in Bristol gathering dust in a museum provided by the Department of Community Medicine. Further work is necessary to pluck the full fruits of the research.

As a result of this work, our firm belief was that painstaking investigation of the facts about home accidents was the essential pre-requisite for health education programmes on safety. Facts must be established before effective safety measures can be designed. For example, there is no point in running an amnesty campaign to get grannies to turn in old, unwanted drugs to save the lives of children who might consume them, if few accidents involve old drugs and if the programme itself brings drugs out into the open to be seen and taken by children who otherwise would have ignored them (Calnan, Dale, and de Fonseka, 1976). Or, to take another example, there is little point in making cost-effectiveness studies on how to maximise the exposure of television audiences to a short film about the dangers of saucepans of boiling water, if it is not saucepans but kettles which produce the big problem of scalds. This is why we began with the facts of accidents, not the design of posters, in our study for the Health Education Council.

The Uncertainties of Research and Development

Somewhere back in 1972 or 1973 (the exact date is recorded but lost in the research museum in Bristol), three of us visited an important government department. Once there, we presented the officials with evidence of the incidence of accidents involving kettles: 27 per 100,000 population per year, no fewer than 69 in our studies in Bristol. We had found that most involved kettles that were dropped or knocked over, with the largest proportion of water spilling from under the lid and the spout. We set out provisional details for a safer kettle, that is one that would be proof against domestic accident, error, negligence and even strife, one that would spill no water if it were dropped, knocked, pulled over or even thrown. RoSPA published an article. The data were presented nationally and internationally at scientific meetings.

Twelve months elapsed; an ergonomics research fellow was appointed. He studiously reviewed a variety of projects for safer consumer products involved in accidents we had investigated. He looked at food tins, chip pans, do-it-yourself knives and other products. Improved design of kettles looked most likely to prevent accidents. A designer was appointed. Some prototype kettles were produced at such great cost that it was considered too expensive to put them through the drop test essential to the development programme. Today in 1976, some four to five years later, no safer kettles have come on the market and it is unlikely that any accidents have been prevented as a result of this promising idea; and many thousands of pounds have been spent on this one research and development project on kettles.

Prevention programmes are becoming more prevalent and are based increasingly on good data, good ergonomic ideas, good design, experimental method and government backing. But it is not easy to prevent accidents and, although scientific methods of doing so are continually being investigated, much of the work is likely to be slow and replete with false alleys and failures.

The Bristol studies have shown that some £100,000 invested in research and some 40-50 man-years of study may begin to open up the field. Large-scale research is often essential: take the example of falls. The most frequent problems by far are falls involving stairs, floor surfaces, footwear and a host of environmental and clinical factors. Many means of attack may be necessary to reduce this problem: the use of medilog analysis, falls clinics for the elderly, screening to find Sheldon's drop attack group, alcohol, diuretics and carbon monoxide, as well as architectural, ergonomic and other studies on-site and with the victim of accidents subjected to a list of behavioural and clinical tests. No amount of regular statistics, exchange of information with local enforcement authorities, information from industry about new product hazards as they arise, and exchange of statistical information with other countries is likely to get adequate results in dealing with this problem. So on falls, the biggest single group of accidents in the home, the government document is wide of the mark. Medically based in-depth studies of the kind probably only the Medical Research Council is equipped to pursue are necessary, but will not be sufficient to solve the problem because of the many factors involved. A multi-disciplinary team approach involving many departments is essential to explore such classes of accidents, and these studies must be linked to an epidemiological base to ensure that we can relate the findings back to the community where the accidents happen.

Laboratory Studies and Field Trials

The next stage is the laboratory testing of hypotheses. After this comes the development of prototype environmental and clinical régimes, for example, to reduce the risks of falls or the severity of injury. Next is the development of community-based field trials in which very large numbers of people are equipped with the safer system. The falls of the elderly provide a good example. A large number of the elderly fall when getting in and out of bed or when moving from a chair to a standing position. The incidence of falls may be controlled to some extent by clinical means and better instruction about how and when to take pills, but there will still be many falls. In just the same way that we recommend seat belts to minimise injuries in car accidents because we cannot prevent all car crashes, so we must critically examine the environment of our homes and of our institutions for the care of the elderly and of the young. Is it sane to have concrete floors? Would it be better to have cushion floors? How much cushioning is necessary? Would the necessary safety factors actually precipitate falls? We do not know, since nobody has yet done the necessary experiments. Local Housing Authorities may have the powers to investigate but the DPCP does not. The Building Research Station has the interest and skills for laboratory studies but is probably not equipped for large-scale field trials. It should be, but the consultative document does not seem to cover this very important topic at all, and other examples could be given by matching the points in the document with the league tables of accidents that have been published (Roberts *et al.*, 1974; Dale *et al.*, 1974; USA National Commission on Product Safety, 1970).

Standards

We would now like to refer to the points on standards in the document. The document suggests that ways of speeding up the production of standards might help safety. Our experience is that speed is not the problem, but the system of standards itself. The technical committees of standards organisations are dominated by manufacturers and they do not use the experimental method in setting standards, which are each invented by the relevant committee. At present there is no active work in hand to produce a new standard for steps and ladders in the United Kingdom, yet safer ladders and steps are required and there is inescapable evidence from the field studies of accidents that two types of investigation are necessary for their production: first, human factor analyses of how steps and ladders are used in the domestic environment; and second, experimental studies to produce ladders and steps and test them in the field — this should begin with testing equipment made to a variety of 'safer' designs already available but not considered marketable, or not proven safe.

The National Commission on Product Safety in the United States reprimanded the ladder manufacturers' association there for failing in their duty of research (USA National Commission on Product Safety, 1970). Here we have no commission or bureau with the same powers, and therefore it is essential that proposed legislation makes it a duty for manufacturers, as well as the government where possible, to carry out or sponsor the necessary design research. If this had been done with ladders we might be further forward now. Instead, field research material remains unused for years.

Research Responsibility of Manufacturers

Research by manufacturers, we believe, is a key for future progress in this country. Sections 6 (1) and 6 (2) of the Health and Safety at Work Act 1974 could provide a model for home safety legislation. The first part of section 6 (1) says:

> It shall be the duty of any person who designs, manufactures, imports or supplies any article for use at work — (a) to ensure, so far as is reasonably practicable, that the article is so designed and constructed as to be safe and without risks to health when properly used; (b) to carry out or arrange for the carrying out of such testing and examination as may be necessary for the performance of the duty imposed on him by the preceding paragraph;

and in section 6 (2) the duty is extended in the following way for designers and manufacturers (but not the suppliers or importers):

> to carry out or arrange for the carrying out of any necessary research with a view to the discovery and, so far as is reasonably practicable, the elimination or minimisation of any risks to health or safety to which the design or article may give rise.

This last paragraph, we believe, is one of the most important principles in the Act. Note that it says, 'the elimination or minimisation of any risks to health or safety to which the design or article *may give rise*' so the research is not to be limited to accidents and occasions of risk when the manufacturer considers that the article was being *properly* used, but is to cover *any risk to health or safety to which the design may give rise.*

This standard of research and safety is provided for articles used at work — and work is defined in section 52 (1) as 'work as an employee or as a self-employed person', with these terms in turn defined to exclude those who do unpaid work at home for themselves and their families. Yet the place of work of nearly half the adult population of this country is in the home, and since most of them are not employed or self-employed within the terms of the Act, they are not afforded the protection of the Act. At work, within the meaning of the given definition, 1,000 people are killed each year; almost 7,000 people are killed in a year in homes in the United Kingdom. The standard of research required in sections 6 (1) and 6 (2) of the Health and Safety at Work Act should be equally applicable to home safety and should be included in future legislation on that subject.

Foolproof Equipment

In hospitals we have three standards for equipment in ascending order of safety; safe, foolproof and nurseproof. Section 1 (9) of the consultative document suggests that 'consumer-proof' against all foreseeable misuse is too high a standard for households. We beg to differ.

In Section 4 (109) of the document this theme of the foolhardy person in the community is again considered. The document asserts: 'It is not possible by legislative means to prevent the foolhardy from exposing themselves and their families to unnecessary risks.' This bland assertion denies a century of experience in public health and indeed the very basis for much of our transport safety controls. It used to be claimed that no one need die from drinking fetid water: you could either boil it after getting it from the pump or not drink it at all. It is similarly claimed by some that dental health is a matter of education, tooth brushing and the use of fluoride tablets. The history of public health tells us that the legislation for the arterial system of water supply, chlorination and now fluoridation is necessary to protect the foolhardy from themselves. Indeed, much of the existing industrial safety legislation was built on the assumption that legislation is necessary to save the blind, infants, those too old, too ill or too foolish to learn for themselves from the worst effects of their freedom of action and that of their neighbours. We also know from experience that even the most prudent consumer is at times foolhardy, blind or foolish. It is an inescapable fact of human nature. We must design with this in mind.

Health Education

It may be cheap merely to mount campaigns to try to persuade the consumer to be safe in his ways, but do such campaigns work? The primary targets for health education on home safety are not so much the consumer and the general public as manufacturers, retailers, councillors, Health Authorities, the Gas Board, the Electricity Board, the other giant public industries and the legislators themselves. On home safety education the consultative document is too limited in its approach.[4] We have to turn to road safety for an example of health education facing a national accident problem with appropriate fearless realism. The objective of the education programme on seat belts has been unequivocally to achieve and demonstrate sufficient public support to make compulsion by legislation acceptable to the legislators and to the police. We must demand a fearless realism from those directing efforts on home safety who must not be diverted from their course if the Gas Board, the Electricity Board, housing authorities or the government itself are to be the targets for education.

The Last Decade and the Next

The title we have chosen for this somewhat discursive paper is 'A Critical Review of the 1976 Government Consultative Document on Consumer Safety' and it may appear that the criticism has been strong and the review inadequate to cover the full scope of the consultative document. However, in conclusion, we would like to stress that it was a welcome surprise to read that the Department has responded so positively to the obvious need for action and legislation. We are sure that researchers in this country greeted with enthusiasm the publication of the consultative document. We should be less than honest if we were to deny our pleasure in seeing the battle for domestic safety now being joined by the big battalions on the side of action based on data and of epidemiological systems.

E. M. Backett (1965) wrote just over ten years ago in his seminal work on domestic accidents for the World Health Organisation:

> The home is traditionally a stronghold rarely invaded by legislation and in consequence . . . its occupants remain substantially unprotected by the law . . . Much of the existing literature [on domestic accidents] lacks clarity, definitions are elusive and the recognition of the multitude of variables involved has obviously deterred many serious research workers . . . Irritating or futile exhortations to be careful and a mass of ill-focused and sometimes costly propaganda inevitably results, but even this is hardly ever evaluated . . . [which has] gone a long way to render the subject beneath the dignity of epidemiologists and research workers . . . Research in the field [of risk taking] is long overdue and might well claim priority over the floods of consumer research and attitude surveys that are so often produced by able social scientists interested in learning and behaviour changes . . . Systematic review of accident hazards in a sample of households by a team composed of a physician, an engineer and . . . a social scientist, is rarely attempted.

That was Backett's view in 1965, just over ten years ago. In June 1976 we stand inheritors of a decade of progress in just the kind of research prescribed by Professor Backett: systematic, on-site investigations of accidents in the home have increasingly replaced armchair theorising. The major pieces of the puzzle are falling into place. With goodwill, we can take the useful proposals of this consultative document and devise other ways to supplement it in order to establish a scientific basis for home and product safety and for accident control. But this will succeed only if we recall that science is nothing unless based on experimental evidence rather than Socratic enquiry. Epidemiology is interesting but it is not a sufficient basis for national action. In the next decade laboratory experiment and field trials sponsored by the government in a wide range of departments, by the Medical Research Council, and by industry must develop from the work done by the field epidemiology of the last decade. The evidence of accidents and the proofs of lack of safety are not to be found in the casualty department or on the post-mortem table; they are to be traced at the scene of the injury. And that is where the experiments to increase safety in the home must ultimately take place.

Notes

1. This problem was the subject of detailed study by our Bristol research group (Simpson, Calnan and de Fonseka, 1974).
2. The summary of the government consultative document is reproduced as an appendix to this paper.
3. Dr J. W. Dale was director of the Division, Dr C. P. de Fonseka was the designer and first co-ordinator of the project; Dr J. L. Roberts was co-ordinator of the project after 1972; Mr Michael Calnan, a sociologist, now with National Children's Bureau, Mr Don Simpson, a systems analyst and gas chemist now with Avon Health Authority, Mrs Heather Whicher, a barrister, Mr Peter Wood, an ergonomist and Mr Malcolm Lord, a glass technologist, also worked with us on the project.
4. The consultative document concentrates only on the need for home safety education of the consumer.

References

Backett, E. M. (1965) *Domestic Accidents* (Public Health Papers No. 26). Geneva: World Health Organisation.

Calnan, M., Dale, J. W., and de Fonseka, C. P. (1976) Suspected poisoning in children. *Archives of Disease in Childhood* 51, 180-5.

Dale, J. W., Roberts, J. L., de Fonseka, C. P., Simpson, D., Knight, M. and Payne, V. (1974) Home Accidents and Health Education Investments. NATO Symposium on Working Place Safety, Proceedings, Bad Grund, Federal Republic of Germany. Mimeo.

Department of Prices and Consumer Protection (1976a) *Collection of information on accidents in the home*. London: DPCP.

Department of Prices and Consumer Protection (1976b) *Consumer Safety. A Consultative Document*. Cmnd, 6398. London: HMSO.

Gill, C. (August, 1973) Step Ladders. *Handyman Which?* 113-19. London: Consumer's Association.

Lord, G. M. (1974) A Provisional Review of home accidents involving flat glass in North East Bristol. Joint study by Pilkington Bros. Ltd. and the Bristol Medical Research Division of the Health Education Council. Mimeo.

Roberts, J. L., Payne, V., Dale, J. W., Northover, D., Simmons, L. and de Fonseka, C. P. (1974) Home Accidents and health education. *Health Education Journal* 33, No. 2, 35-45, and No. 3, 67-78.

Simpson, D., Calnan, M. and de Fonseka, C. P. (1974) Factors contributing to bathroom accidents from carbon monoxide poisoning. *Community Health* 5, 271-7.

Slater, J. (1973) *An Accidental Death*. Granada Television UK. 16mm sound colour film. Manchester: Granada F.T. Film Library.

USA National Commission on Product Safety (1970) *Hearings of the Commission*, Vols. 1-10, and *Final Report*. New York: Law-Art Publishers.

Yeats, K., Roberts, J. L. and Dale, J. W. (1974) Health Education and Kettle Accidents — Report. Bristol: Medical Research Division, Health Education Council. Mimeo.

APPENDIX: EXTRACT FROM GOVERNMENT CONSULTATIVE DOCUMENT ON CONSUMER SAFETY, 1976*

SECTION V – SUMMARY OF POINTS FOR CONSULTATION

115. Possible changes in the present law and practice discussed in this paper are summarised in the following paragraphs. The proposals and other issues discussed fall into three categories:

    (i)   those on which work has started – paragraph 116;

    (ii)   those where it is suggested that no change should be made – paragraph 117; and

    (iii)   those for consideration – paragraph 118.

Comments on all the proposals, and on any other aspect of the subject, will, however, be taken fully into account in determining future action in this field.

Proposals on which work has started

116. (i) *Data collection:* it is intended to set up a system to provide regular statistics on product-related and other home accidents (paragraph 48).

    (ii)   *In-depth studies:* it is intended to set up a system for carrying out in-depth investigations in selected categories of home accident as part of the accident surveillance system (paragraph 49).

    (iii)   *Liaison with local authorities:* steps are being taken to strengthen channels of communication with local authorities (paragraph 52).

    (iv)   *Exchange of information with other countries:* it is intended to seek and develop contacts with other countries for exchange of information on consumer safety matters (paragraph 57).

    (v)   *Codes of Conduct:* OFT is prepared to include safety requirements in any codes of conduct which it sponsors and in appropriate cases DPCP will itself encourage industries to draw up safety codes in the absence of regulations (paragraph 61).

Issues where it is suggested no change should be made

117. (i) *Consultation prior to making regulations:* no change is proposed in the present consultation pricess preceding the making

---

* Cmnd 6398 *Consumer Safety*

of regulations (paragraph 63).

(ii)   *Private transactions:* it is not proposed that sales by private persons should be brought under control (paragraph 75).

(iii)   *Misuse:* it is proposed to continue to seek requirements in standards and regulations that take account of common misuses revealed by experience, but it is not considered practicable to impose any general obligation on manufacturers to take account of all foreseeable misuses (paragraph 92).

Issues put forward for consideration

118.   Comments and views are invited on the following matters:

(i)   *Notification of hazards by industry:* whether arrangements should be introduced under which manufacturers, importers and distributors would notify to DPCP information about potential hazards in products supplied by them for sale to the general public, and if so what those arrangements should cover and whether they should be statutory (paragraph 54).

(ii)   *Disclosure of information by industry:* whether powers should be sought to obtain on request information relating to product safety from manufacturers, importers and distributors and to require by regulation, where necessary, the provision of such information on any description of products that may be specified, and what provision should be made for information held in confidence (paragraph 56).

(iii)   *Standards:* (a) means of speeding up the writing of standards (paragraph 59) and (b) the existing machinery for the production of international standards (paragraph 60).

(iv)   *Labelling:* whether an extension of the present power should be sought to enable the Secretary of State, by regulation, to prescribe such labelling requirements as appear requisite in any particular case (paragraph 64).

(v)   *Inherently dangerous products:* whether power should be sought to enable the Secretary of State to prohibit outright the sale of any prescribed class of goods where it is considered necessary on grounds of safety and what safeguards would be needed (paragraph 65).

(vi)   *Minimum age of purchase:* whether power should be sought enabling the Secretary of State, by regulation, to prohibit the sale of goods of any description to children below the age specified in the regulation where it is considered necessary on grounds of safety (paragraph 67).

(vii) *References to standards recognised as satisfying regulations:* whether amendment of the Act should be sought to permit regulations to include references to British and international standards conformity with which is not in itself mandatory but is recognised as satisfying the regulations (paragraph 68).

(viii) *Revision of standards referred to in regulations:* whether it is desirable to seek power to provide in regulations that reference to a specified standard may operate as a reference to that standard as currently in force (paragraph 69).

(ix) *Prior approval and certification marks:* whether power should be sought to enable the Secretary of State (a) to impose, by regulation, requirements by reference to certification by any specified body; and (b) to confer such recognition as may be considered appropriate in any particular case on the marks or certificates of conformity issued by certification bodies (paragraph 71).

(x) *Tests to be made during manufacture:* whether powers should be sought to enable the Secretary of State, by regulation, to prescribe requirements as to tests to be made during the manufacture of any prescribed class of consumer goods where these may be relevant to the safety of the end product (paragraph 72).

(xi) *Safety equipment:* whether an extension of the present powers should be sought to enable requirements to be imposed relating to the efficiency of safety equipment (paragraph 73).

(xii) *Transactions other than by sale:* whether an extension of the Act should be sought to cover any goods supplied in the course of a business (paragraph 74).

(xiii) *Jumble sales, etc.:* whether goods sold at jumble sales, sales of work and like functions should remain outside the scope of new consumer safety legislation (paragraph 75).

(xiv) *Prohibition of manufacture or importation of goods which do not comply with regulations:* whether powers to prohibit, by regulation, the manufacture or import of goods which do not comply with regulations are desirable and practicable (paragraph 76).

(xv) *Servicing:* whether new legislation should make provision for the prescription, by regulation, of such safety requirements affecting servicing as may be appropriate for any class of goods (paragraph 78).

(xvi) *General prohibition on sale of unsafe goods and on unsafe servicing:* whether new legislation should make it an offence for any manufacturer, importer or trader not to exercise due care to satisfy himself that the goods he supplies are safe when properly used for their intended purpose, or that any servicing he carries out on any goods does not render those goods unsafe (paragraph 84).

(xvii) *Banning orders:* whether power should be sought to enable the Secretary of State, by order, to ban the sale of any named product or description of goods where this appears necessary on grounds of safety (paragraph 89).

(xviii) *Duty of enforcement:* whether local weights and measures authorities' responsibility for enforcing consumer safety legislation should be made mandatory (paragraph 93).

(xix) *Seizure and destruction of dangerous goods:* whether there is sufficient evidence to justify enforcement authorities being empowered to seize goods which do not comply with regulations (or banning orders) if this seems expedient in the interests of public safety, and what constraints should be imposed on the exercise of any such powers (paragraph 95).

(xx) *Recall of unsafe goods:* whether there should be powers to require anyone who has supplied dangerous goods to take the necessary steps, at his own expense, to recall them and issue appropriate warnings, and how any such powers might be exercised and enforced (paragraph 98).

(xxi) *Co-ordination of enforcement:* whether machinery to provide greater co-ordination of national enforcement arrangements should be established and, if so, in what form (paragraph 101).

(xxii) *Responsibility for functions:* whether all the functions relevant to regulatory responsibilities, including central collection and evaluation of information concerning consumer safety, should continue to be the responsibility of DPCP (paragraph 104).

(xxiii) *Publicity and education:* how effective present publicity and education activities are in reducing product-related and other home accidents and in encouraging greater care on the part of consumers (paragraph 114).

Submission of views

119. Written comments on any or all of the proposals outlined in this paper together with any other views on the subject should be sent by 31 May 1976 to the Department of Prices and Consumer Protection, Fair Trading Division (Consumer Safety Unit), Room 412, 1 Victoria Street, London, SW1H 0ET.

6 SOME SOCIAL AND LEGAL CONSEQUENCES OF ACCIDENTS IN THE HOME

H. G. Genn and S. B. Burman

Introduction

The Centre for Socio-Legal Studies is currently engaged in a group of research projects concerned with compensation and support for victims of 'misfortune'. The broad aim of these studies is to investigate the social, economic and legal consequences of serious functional difficulties arising from injury, illness and handicap. The research is concerned with changes in people's lives (whether permanent or temporary) of a social and economic kind, and the ways in which victims and their families cope with such unexpected changes in normal living. We are attempting to assess the number of people in the general population whose activities are limited as a result of these kinds of misfortune and to identify in some detail the problems and needs which arise as a result of such limitations. An integral part of the work involves a critical examination of the range of compensatory systems which exist to support such victims and the extent to which these systems meet or fail to meet the needs of victims. We have focused particularly on the legal system, the income maintenance system, local authority welfare services and informal systems of support.

The central part of the project involves a national household survey, in which 15,000 households are being screened for cases of functional interruption resulting from accidents, illness or congenital disability. This screening operation is designed to produce nationally representative incidence data on functional limitations resulting from such causes, and to supply samples of victims who have suffered road accidents, work accidents, domestic accidents and assault, as well as cases of chonic and acute sickness, for further detailed study at a second stage of the research.

Pilot Survey on Home Accidents

As part of the preliminary work on this national survey a pilot study of home accident victims was carried out in Bristol in 1974. This survey had two major objectives: first, to obtain a sample of people who had suffered 'serious' functional interruptions as a result of an accident in the home and to pilot questions concerning the social and economic consequences for the victim which resulted from the accident; and second, to investigate the extent to which the victims of these accidents made use of the legal process to recover compensation for their injuries.

To achieve these objectives the study was devised in two stages. The first stage consisted of a screening operation conducted by post which would identify those victims who satisfied our criteria for further study. The second stage involved the administration of a structured questionnaire to victims (or their parents in the case of victims under fourteen) who had been screened out on the basis of their answers to the postal questionnaire. Victims were included in the second stage of the study if they had either suffered serious injury in the home accident, or if they blamed another person (other than a family member) for their accident; or, finally, if they satisfied both of these criteria.

Our definition of 'serious' injury was not based on any clinical diagnosis of injuries suffered, but on the extent to which victims had been unable to carry out their normal activities as a result of the injuries. This definition of seriousness is derived from the hypothesis that, irrespective of actual injury, the inability to function normally implies a degree of dependence on others. We were interested in the ways in which different people overcame such difficulties, the range of informal networks of support and the differing access to such systems for victims, as well as the use made of official supporting agencies. Consequently this criterion for inclusion in the second stage of the study rested not on a description of the injuries suffered in the accident, but on whether victims had been unable to carry out normally one or more 'key' activities for a period of three weeks or more. These key activities were in the areas of self-care, mobility, employment, housework and communication.[1] The genesis of the second criterion for inclusion in the study – whether or not the victim blamed a third party for the accident– is a little more complicated. It is related to the legal provision for compensation and is explained in detail in the section on the use of legal services.

Our original sample of victims was obtained from the Medical Research Division of the Health Education Council,[2] which conducted a survey of home accidents in Bristol from 1970 to 1975. A home accident was defined as 'an unpleasant, unexpected and unwanted occurrence in a chain of physical events within the domestic home and garden which resulted in either bodily harm or material damage or both'. Certain categories of accidents were excluded, namely accidents

to people visiting homes, those which happened to people who were in
homes only in the course of paid employment, and accidents in
residential institutions, hotels and boarding houses.

The area selected for the Health Education Council study was
formed from nine contiguous electoral wards in north east Bristol,
which included decaying nineteenth-century inner parts of the city,
industrial suburbs, enveloped villages, ribbon developments along the
arterial roads and new housing estates. The Medical Research Division
collected cases over five separate periods, and for the purposes of our
study we used the cases of personal injury collected in the last period,
from November 1972 to June 1973. A description of the manner in
which the sample was collected appears in the preceding paper by Dr
J. L. Roberts and Dr J. W. Dale. Our sample consisted of 1,234
accidents, involving 1,214 people (20 of whom had suffered two
accidents during the period) of which 457 (38 per cent) were under the
age of 15 at the time of the accident. A short screening questionnaire
was sent to all of these 1,234 cases asking whether the accident
which the victim had suffered had resulted in any difficulty in carrying
out our 'key' activities; and whether they thought that any of a given
list of people had been wholly or partly to blame for their accident.

Of the 1,234 questionnaires posted, 871 (71 per cent) produced
some response and 798 answered the questionnaire fully. Of the 871
questionnaires returned, 175 cases (20 per cent) claimed that their
injury had caused an interruption of three weeks or more in at least
one of the listed activities. Of the 871 cases, 64 (7 per cent) claimed
that someone else, other than a family member, was at least partly to
blame for their accident. Of these 64, 18 victims had also suffered
some activity interruption of three weeks or more. Thus our second
stage sample consisted of 221 victims who satisfied one or both of the
screening criteria.

For this second stage a structured questionnaire, administered by
an interviewer, had been devised. Questions were asked on a number
of topics including medical data, employment and income data, as well
as questions about the use of the legal system to obtain compensation
for injuries, and information about the nature of formal and informal
support received after the accident. By the time fieldwork had been
completed we had obtained interviews with 127 victims who had
suffered functional interruptions for the specified length of time, and
44 interviews with victims who had not suffered a long interruption of
normal activities but who blamed a third party for their accident.

The group of victims who had suffered long interruptions of normal

activities was composed primarily of women (77 per cent) and biased
towards the older age groups. A third of the sample were aged over
65, and a further third were in the 50-65 age category. A high proportion of these victims lived in one- or two-person households, often
where there was no wage-earner present (see Table 1)

Table 1 Number of Persons in Employment Compared with Number of
Persons in Household

No. in household in employment		No. of persons in household							TOTAL	%
		1	2	3	4	5	6	7+		
None	%	40.8	36.7	12.2	8.2	2.0	0.0	0.0	100.0	
	n.	20	18	6	4	1	0	0	49	38.6
One	%	0.0	42.3	15.4	13.5	15.4	0.0	13.5	100.0	
	n.	0	22	8	7	8	0	7	52	40.9
Two	%	0.0	20.0	25.0	25.0	25.0	5.0	0.0	100.0	
	n.	0	4	5	5	5	1	0	20	15.7
Three+	%	0.0	0.0	16.7	16.7	50.0	0.0	16.7	100.0	
	n.	0	0	1	1	3	0	1	6	4.8
TOTAL	%	15.7	34.6	15.7	13.4	13.4	0.8	6.3	100.0	
	n.	20	44	20	17	17	1	8	127	100.0

All of the twenty single-person households consisted of people of age
60 and over, and exactly three-quarters of the two-person households
were couples both aged over 60. The age, sex and residence pattern of
this sample was very different from that of the population at large, and
is explicable and consistent with expectations in that those people
most at risk of suffering an accident in the home are elderly women
who might normally reside in single-person or small households.

According to the medically-based criteria used by the Health Education
Council, the most common injuries suffered by this sample were
fractures of upper limbs, severe fractures of lower limbs and minor
lacerations of upper limbs. Of the 127 injuries coded, just under a
quarter were 'severe', just over two-fifths were 'moderate', and a
third were 'minor' injuries. These injuries were caused most frequently
by falls, collisions, and burning (both by liquids and appliances)

(see Table 2).

Table 2 Distribution of Injury Type and Body Area Affected in Victim Sample

TYPE OF INJURY n = 127		AFFECTED BODY AREA n = 127	
Fracture	37.8	Upper limbs	40.9
Laceration	29.9	Lower limbs	36.2
Sprain	15.7	Whole body	7.9
Burns, scald	12.6	Head	4.7
Dislocation	2.4	Chest	3.9
Concussion	1.6	Abdomen	2.4
		Spine	1.6
		Pelvis/buttocks	1.6
		Neck	.8

Respondents were asked whether they had been to hospital within 24 hours of the accident: 62 per cent had visited hospital but had not been detained, 14 per cent had stayed overnight, 7 per cent had been admitted for between four days and three weeks and 5 per cent had remained in hospital for between one and six months. Twelve per cent of victims had not been to hospital at all.[3] Three-quarters of all victims had attended out-patients' clinics and half of this number had attended on a weekly or more frequent basis. Of those attending an out-patients' clinic, 17 per cent attended once only, 31 per cent attended for up to four weeks and 38 per cent attended for between one and six months. Seven victims (8 per cent) actually attended an out-patients' clinic for more than six months. The number of victims who saw their own general practitioner following the accident was similar to the number attending hospital. In all, 62 per cent saw their doctor after the accident and mainly on one occasion only (29 per cent), although 19 per cent (14 victims) claimed to have seen him nine times or more as a result of the accident. As might be expected, victims in the older age groups were detained in hospital more frequently than younger victims and for longer periods of time, but no statistical tests showed this trend to be significant.

The most common activity problems suffered by victims following the accident were washing, and those activities involving mobility; although amongst women living alone a very high proportion had difficulty with the major housework tasks (see Table 3).

Table 3 Relative Frequencies of Activity Limitation among Victim Sample (n = 127)

Washing	59.0
Walking	58.2
Climbing	57.3
Taking the bus	52.7
Shopping	47.9
Cleaning	47.3
Washing Clothes	46.3
Cooking	40.0
Using WC	30.6
Working	25.2
Eating	20.5
Working full-time	15.8
School activities	9.5
Going to school	7.0
Talking	2.3

Table 4 shows the lengths of time for which victims were unable to carry out particular activities, and from this it can be seen that for many victims, the period of interruption in normal functioning was quite long.

A number of people were still suffering from the effects of the accident at the time of the interview, which took place up to 18 months later. Some 43 per cent of victims claimed that they were still suffering some ill effects from their accident. Of these 54 victims, 35 said that they did not expect any improvement in their condition in the near future (65 per cent) and six victims said that they did not know whether their condition would improve.

Respondents characteristically suffered from a combination of activity limitation following their accident, rather than simply a single difficulty. The distribution of number of activity limitations by age was, perhaps surprisingly, not significant, although as age increased there was a slight tendency for the number of activity limitations

Table 4 Period of Interruption in Carrying out Normal Activities Among Victim Sample

	Up to 3 weeks %	1-6 months %	More than 6 months %	Total %	Total n
Washing	52	39	9	100	75
Using WC	51	33	15	100	39
Eating	46	38	15	100	26
Climbing stairs	38	38	23	100	73
Walking	50	27	23	100	74
Using the bus	42	28	30	100	67
Shopping	42	33	25	100	61
Cleaning	47	30	23	100	60
Cooking	49	29	21	100	51
Washing clothes	44	36	20	100	59
Going to work	25	56	19	100	32
Going to school	55	44	–	100	9

suffered to increase. This was most marked for the 51-70 age group.

Informal Support and Local Authority Service Use

We know from published sources that the proportion of the population which actually makes use of the available local authority support services is relatively small when taking into account the range of contingencies which might result in the need for assistance in a family. We were interested in the kinds of help people received from informal sources in a time of 'crisis', such as an incapacitating injury. To obtain some idea of the kinds of informal help received following the accident and resultant difficulties with normal functioning, all respondents were asked whether they had received any help in taking care of themselves, doing housework or moving around after the accident, and, if so, who had provided this help and for what period of time. Over three-quarters of victims had received help in one or more areas of activity and, of these, just over a fifth had received help with more than five different activities. The activities for which help was most frequently received were shopping, washing and dressing, and washing clothes. The need for assistance was spread across all age groups, although the proportion of victims receiving this kind of assistance was somewhat higher in the over-50 age groups. We found that, in general, spouses and children gave assistance most frequently, but that the use of informal support from outside the home (i.e. neighbours, friends and other relatives) increased for housework activities such as cooking, cleaning, and shopping (see Figure 1). All functions, both personal and household, were performed with the help of informal sources for fairly long periods. For nearly every activity mentioned, approximately half of the assistance received was for more than one month. Thus it appears that this kind of informal help is undertaken as a fairly lengthy commitment and not necessarily as a short-term expedient.

In order to investigate the degree of use made of local authority services among our victim population, respondents were given a show card on which was printed a list of local authority services and were asked whether they had made any use of the services following their accident. From this we found that sixteen respondents (13 per cent) had used home helps; nine respondents had used meals on wheels (7 per cent); and one or two had seen social workers and made use of day centres. Three-quarters of those making use of home helps were still receiving this aid at the time of the interview. Of those respondents who had used meals on wheels, only a third were still receiving them

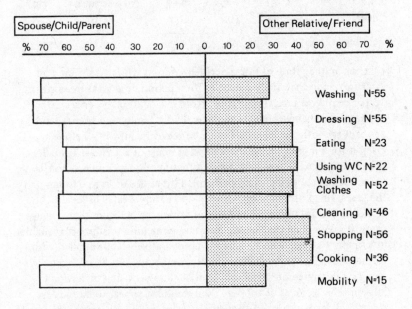

Figure 1 Identity of Those Giving Informal Assistance

at the time of the interview. In general we found that those people
who made use of home helps tended also to receive meals on wheels,
and overall use of such services was predominantly by those in the over-
60 age group. From the data which we received on the questionnaire
it is apparent that help from local authorities was generally used *in
addition* to informal assistance, since the majority of victims using local
authority services were already getting some sort of help from family
and friends before the accident. It was very rare to find a victim who
received no help from informal sources at all and was supported
entirely by official services (see Table 5).

Table 5 Use of Informal Support by Use of Local Authority Services

INFORMAL SUPPORT	FORMAL SUPPORT					
	Yes		No		Total	
	%	n.	%	n.	%	n.
Yes	14.1	(14)	85.8	(85)	100.0	(99)
No	7.1	(2)	92.8	(26)	100.0	(28)
Total	12.6	(16)	87.4	(111)	100.0	(127)

Thus, in the group of home accident victims who had suffered an
interruption in their daily activities for a period of at least three weeks,
12 per cent were receiving support from local authority services, 78
per cent were being supported informally by family and friends, and 11
per cent by both. At least half of those receiving informal help were
given it for a month or more over a wide range of activities. Though
personal tasks were generally assisted by household members, household
tasks, such as shopping, were performed by outsiders in more than half
the cases. In comparison with Bristol and national rates of local
authority service use, members of our sample were higher than average
users. It seems then that we are examining the kind of support available
informally to those who are already comparatively well supplied with
formal sources of support. The study group could not be said to be
seeking to compensate for a low level of state provision by having to
rely on other sources of support. Neither did it appear to be the case
that a high level of local authority provision was encouraging individuals
to rely solely on the state, allowing families to avoid their responsibilities.

In fact, high levels of both formal and informal support appear to go together, though informal support is available to a much larger population.

Those respondents who had not used any local authority services were asked, for each service listed on a show card, whether or not they had heard of the service and if so whether they had ever made an application to receive it. Where a victim claimed to know about a particular service but had not applied for it, they were asked why they had not applied. We found that among those respondents who claimed to have knowledge of the services listed, the expressed reasons for not having made any use of such services fell mainly into the categories of 'I didn't need it', 'the family could cope', and 'I didn't know I was eligible'.

The response 'I didn't need it' as a reason for not applying covers a multitude of ambiguities. It seems that this category of response might contain three types of people: first, those who objectively probably would not have needed any help from anyone, since their activity limitation could be overcome personally (i.e. those victims who could manage certain things with difficulty alone but who did not find that there was anything which they could not do at all); second, those victims who felt that they did not need help because they had mobilised informal help from family and friends, but did not state this fact specifically; and third, those people who regard Local Authority services as a 'charity' intended for people 'worse off' than themselves (although objectively they might have appeared to have been in need of some assistance), and regard it as demeaning to accept official help.

It is impossible to make any judgement on the basis of the questions as to whether or not those respondents who did not think they were eligible for help would in fact have received any had they applied to a local authority. It is nevertheless interesting that a not insignificant minority of victims were under the impression that local authorities required certain qualifications before their help would be forthcoming, and it would be interesting to investigate this point further. The number of victims who said that they had not applied because their families could cope with the problem clearly illustrates the extent to which individuals seem to look upon the social services as a 'last resort' when all other informal methods of overcoming difficulties have been exhausted or are not forthcoming.

Employment and Income Data

This section of the questionnaire was concerned with questions about the effects of the accident in relation to employment and household income. As we have already noted, our sample was composed mainly of elderly women and thus questions relating to employment and loss of income were not often relevant to respondents. In addition, we encountered some response problems in this section, which limited the amount of data recorded. All respondents over the age of sixteen were asked what their job had been at the time of the accident and what their usual income had been at that time. Only 30.7 per cent (39) of the sample had been employed at the time of the accident and, of these people, only 28 respondents gave any information about what their income had been. Thirty-three victims had taken time off work as a result of the accident and 25 of these had been off for one month or more (76 per cent). Of the 33 respondents who claimed to have taken time off work, only 9 (27 per cent) stated that they had received their normal income during this period. Six respondents claimed to have changed their job as a result of the accident and 20 victims (16 per cent) said that other people in their family had taken time off work as a result of the accident. Of the people in the family who took time off work as a result of the accident, just over a third were off for up to three days; 55 per cent were off for between four days and three weeks and 10 per cent had time off work amounting to between one and six months. Two fifths of those taking time off were spouses; two fifths were children; and the remaining fifth were other relatives. No victim reported that any family member was obliged to change his job as a result of the victim's accident.

In addition we were interested to discover whether the accident had resulted in a reduction in available income by indirect means, such as extra expenditure resulting from the accident. Some of the victims (9 per cent) claimed to have had extra laundry costs; 6 per cent had extra clothing and heating costs; 5 per cent had extra transport costs and 3 per cent had to spend more on food. Sixteen per cent of victims claimed to have spent their savings as a result of the accident (20 people). For some people it was necessary to draw out savings merely to cover the cost of normal living expenses (7 people). Others used savings for special purposes related to the accident. One family reported, for example:

> [We] spent from savings to put mother in a home for three weeks so that we could go on holiday. [We] paid £20 of the £45-50 which

it cost, from savings.

Or, for example, a victim reported: '[I] spent from savings to pay a woman to come in and do the housework.'

It appears then that among this group of home accident victims the injuries suffered resulted in a considerable amount of time being taken off work, both by the victims themselves and occasionally by other family members. Losses in household income were experienced by victims directly as a result of time taken off work and extra expenditure on both goods and services also reduced money available to the household.

Use of Legal Services

In order to place in perspective our study of the use of legal services by home accident victims, it is necessary first to outline briefly the provisions made by law for compensating victims of personal injury. Apart from benefits paid to certain categories of victim by the welfare state, the most important method of obtaining compensation for injury is through the tort system of the common law (the rules laid down by the judges). Under this process, compensation for death or injury suffered in accidents can be awarded by a judge against a third party whose fault directly caused the accident. Thus, if a victim can prove that his injury resulted from the negligence of another person, he may recover compensation from that person. In common law it is not sufficient merely to have suffered injury in an accident to be eligible for compensation, but it must be shown that some person was legally responsible for the accident. In this way the *needs* of the victim do not represent sufficient grounds for entitlement to compensation. There must be a reason for shifting the loss suffered by the victim to another person held responsible for such losses. If no third party can be held liable in this way, the victim must go uncompensated, bearing his losses alone so far as the common law is concerned.

Thus the tort system at present distinguishes between different categories of accident victim; not on the basis of the injuries suffered and the resulting losses to the individual and his family, but on whether or not another person caused the accident. A victim who suffers paralysis after being knocked down by a car may be eligible for compensation while a victim who suffers the same injury after falling down the stairs in his home probably would not. Regardless of the fact that the consequences for the victims might be very similar in the two cases, eligibility for compensation rests on the nature of the accident and not on its consequences.

For claims which come to court, the amount of damages to be awarded is decided by a judge sitting alone. There is no ceiling fixed for the amount which can be awarded by the judge and payment is made in the form of a single lump sum. The main items for which damages are assessed are: future loss of earnings of the victim (based on an assessment of *post*-accident expectation of life), non-economic losses such as the pain and suffering experienced by the victim as a result of the accident, loss of expectation of life, and loss of the capacity to enjoy life. In the case of death caused by the fault of a third party, the dependents of the victim can claim compensation for their loss of pecuniary benefit from the deceased victim. There is no payment in these cases for relatives' grief or misery, and children do not receive compensation for loss of parental care or affection.

Since most people who are in a position to be held liable to pay damages insure against that risk (for example, motorists, employers and manufacturers), the majority of damages payments are made not by individuals, but by insurance companies. In practice, only a small minority of claims actually come to court to be decided by a judge; the remainder are resolved outside the court (and thus to an extent outside the normal judicial process) on the basis of negotiations betwen between insurance companies and claimants' solicitors.

Home accident victims, then, in common with other accident victims, are free to pursue a claim for compensation through the courts if they can prove that the negligence of a third party caused their accident. If no third party negligence can be shown, there is little chance of financial assistance except from the means-tested Supplementary Benefits scheme. By definition, those people most likely to be injured in a domestic accident are those groups which spend the greater part of their time in the home — the elderly, housewives and children. These are the very groups excluded from most social security provision by virtue of their status as non-earners.

The 'freedom' of home accident victims to pursue a claim in the courts, is, however, apparently exercised relatively infrequently. In 1970, according to official statistics, in England and Wales, 6,463 people died as a result of domestic accidents; 97,620 people were admitted to hospital because of their injuries; and an estimated two million people were involved in accidents in the home which resulted in minor injuries or property damage (Thomson and Hesketh, 1975). The risk to individuals in the under-65 age group of accidental death in the home is as high as between a third and a half of that from death in a road accident (Alphey and Leach, 1974). Despite these statistics, an examination of reported law cases suggests that only a very few victims of domestic accidents claim damages through the legal system, whereas there are many claims by road accident and work accident victims.

There are a number of possible reasons for this difference. First, that fewer home accident victims actually have grounds for legal action under the tort system or that the losses suffered in home accidents are considered too small to warrant instituting legal proceedings. More possibly, victims are simply not aware of their legal rights and fail to think in terms of legal remedies for injuries suffered in accidents in the home. In our pilot study in Bristol we wished to gain some information about why our sample of victims did, or did not, make claims for damages for their injuries. To accomplish this task adequately it would have been necessary to distinguish between those accidents where the victim had at least a *prima facie* case for compensation, and those where there appeared to be no grounds for any legal action. However, given that we were collecting information from questionnaires and not conducting a thorough investigation of accidents, it was not possible to assemble sufficient data to identify those victims who would clearly have had a case against a third party. Since the tort system is based on the blame-worthiness of a third party, we attempted to discover which victims might conceivably have considered claiming compensation by asking victims whether they blamed another person for their accident. This was not a particularly satisfactory criterion, since the concept of blame covers notions of moral blame as well as those more like legal blame, but no more generally intelligible test could be devised.

Respondents were given, on both the postal questionnaire and later at a detailed interview, a list of possible 'blamees' and asked whether they thought that any were responsible for their particular accident. The list contained the following: a shop or manufacturer; a workman, such as a builder or plumber; a local council; a landlord; a neighbour; someone else in the family; any other person; only their own fault; and no one's fault. There was a remarkably high degree of inconsistency between answers to the postal questionnaire and the detailed interview on this point, possibly as a result of respondents confusing the details of different accidents. However, of the minority of respondents who did blame a third party for their accident (18 per cent of all victims answering the postal questionnaire), more than two-thirds claimed that a family member was the person to blame. Of those who mentioned someone other than a family member, a shop or manufacturer was most commonly blamed for the accident, followed by a local council, a landlord, a workman and, finally, neighbours.

In both the postal questionnaire and the follow-up interviews, respondents were asked whether they had thought of trying to claim compensation for their injuries from the people whom they thought were to blame for the accident. Seven people stated on the screening questionnaire that they had considered claiming compensation, of whom only five were available for re-interview, and of those five, only two victims confirmed that they had in fact considered claiming compensation. Thus, together with one woman who changed her answers from negative to positive on this question between the two data collection procedures, we were left with only three victims out of an original total of 871 returned postal questionnaires who had actually considered claiming legal compensation for their injuries. Of these three cases, only two victims finally took legal advice. The third (a victim burnt by oil from a faulty chip pan) did not take advice because the manufacturers of the pan had informed her that 'insurance companies would not accept responsibility for faulty goods.' Of the two who took legal advice, one had dropped her case and the second was not sure at the time of the interview whether or not the case was actually continuing, since she had had no communication with her solicitor for some time.

The one fact which emerges clearly from this pilot study is that regardless of individual case details, not one member of the sample of victims injured in home accidents had come even close to receiving compensation for injuries via the legal system. Whether the problem lies in the ineligibility of victims according to the rules of the law, or whether it is the 'legal ignorance' of victims who might be eligible, or an unwillingness to use the legal system, is, in a sense, immaterial. The inescapable fact is that the tort system provides virtually no response to the needs of such victims. The findings of the study are unlikely to surprise those people with an interest in the present system of compensation for personal injuries. It is not particularly novel to demonstrate that the tort system is in many respects arbitrary, resulting in occasionally generous awards for the minority of cases which survive the hurdles of the legal system but offering little solace for those which fall by the wayside.

The shortcomings of the present system have been officially recognised by the establishment of a Royal Commission on Civil Liability and Compensation for Personal Injury. This Commission *inter alia*

will evaluate the operation of the New Zealand accident compensation
scheme, which came into effect in 1974, some years after the Wood-
house Report in New Zealand on compensation for injury. The New
Zealand scheme represents a radical approach to compensation for
accidental injuries, under which everyone injured in any type of
accident, irrespective of cause, is entitled to claim compensation from
a state agency, the Accident Compensation Commission. Thus, under
this scheme the victims of road traffic accidents, industrial accidents,
domestic, sporting and leisure accidents as well as criminal injuries,
are all entitled to compensation regardless of the specific details relating
to the cause of the accident, its location or timing. Earnings-related
benefits are paid to victims on a weekly basis up to a ceiling of 80 per
cent of the victim's total loss of earnings. In addition, compensation in
the form of lump sums can be awarded for non-economic losses, such
as pain and suffering, loss of amenities, disfigurement, etc. Lump sums
are also paid where an injury involves the permanent loss or impair-
ment of a bodily function or the loss of any part of the body. In the
case of fatal accidents, compensation related to the benefits which the
victim would have received had he survived the injury are paid to the
surviving dependents.

The scheme consists of three main compensation funds: the Earners
Fund, the Motor Vehicle Fund and the Supplementary Compensation
Fund. The first two funds cover all accidents suffered by earners and
all accidents which involve motor vehicles. They have been financed
by diverting the contributions previously made to insurance funds,
such as employers' liability insurance, workers' compensation and
compulsory motor insurance, into the new scheme. The Supplementary
Fund covers anyone injured by accident who falls outside the other
two funds, such as non-earners injured in domestic accidents, and is
financed by general taxation. Since the need to determine fault in the
cause of accidents no longer exists, enormous savings have been made
in the administration of the scheme compared with the cost of the
legal system of compensation (similar to that now prevailing in
England) which preceded it. There is evidence of a growing awareness
on several continents of the need to provide financial assistance for
those who suffer injury as a result of an accident, without requiring
them to prove that it was caused by a third party. The New Zealand
scheme demonstrates that radical reform on a national scale in this
area of social policy is possible.

Conclusions and Limitations of the Study

As we noted above, the major objective of this pilot study was to obtain (by means of a postal screening operation) a sample of home accident victims who had suffered interruptions of normal activities for three weeks or more, and to use this sample to pilot questions about the social and financial consequences of such interruptions. In addition, we attempted to obtain substantive data about the use made of the legal system by these victims to gain compensation for injuries suffered.

Before moving on to a general summary of our findings, we should make explicit some limitations inherent in the nature of the study. First, we were using a sample of victims which had been gathered originally over the two years preceding our study. This must have had an effect on the accuracy of victims' recall, particularly when the injuries suffered were often not very serious and had in some cases been followed in the intervening period by other accidents or illnesses. The study clearly illustrated the problems involved in asking about one particular accident when it may have been followed by a more serious incident or occured in conjunction with a long-standing problem, the consequences of which may have been more severe, or which could not be disentangled from those of the particular accident in question. Since respondents for Stage II interviews were selected on the basis of answers to the screening questionnaire, we found at the time of the personal interview that there was often some confusion over which particular accident was in question. It is in the nature of such retrospective studies that pinpointing the particular event in question is difficult if the occurrence of such events is likely to be frequent. Thus, when respondents answered the postal questionnaire, they selected the accident which they assumed was relevant and not necessarily the event for which we had information from the Medical Research Division. Anticipating this kind of confusion, we gave interviewers a brief description of the particular accident in which we were interested. This resulted in some of the questionnaires produced at Stage II not fulfilling the basic screening criteria, because they described a different accident from that mentioned on the postal questionnaire.

In addition to the problem of respondents' recall over time, it is important to note that our Stage II questionnaire represented at least the third time that respondents had answered questions from researchers about their accident, and this may have caused some respondents to be impatient and perhaps less willing to probe their memories in relation to events immediately following the accident. Given these limitations however, we found that on the whole respondents were interested in the questionnaire and (with the exception of financial questions) were willing to provide the information required.

Although in Stage I of the study we obtained a relatively high response rate to the postal screening questionnaire (70 per cent), the confusion which was exposed when personal interviews were conducted at Stage II leads us to the conclusion that the use of postal question- naires to screen for this kind of sample is not the ideal method. Apart from the problem of confusion over the event in question, our analysis of non-respondents to the postal screen indicated that there was a significant tendency for the more serious cases to respond to postal screening, thus producing a biased picture of the incidence of serious injury.

Information gathered at Stage II of the study has demonstrated that respondents are able to recall details of the consequences of specific accidents over a relatively long period of time. Since we have no way of validating most of the information gathered, it is impossible to say to what extent the data presented represent a true reflection of the problems facing our victims at the time of their accident, nor to what extent the memories of difficulties, described to us some two years later, have been distorted. However, on the questions where we could compare our responses with those gained by the Medical Research Division of the Health Education Council in their original interviews, we have some evidence of consistency of response over time. The Stage II sample of victims screened out by the postal questionnaire was composed in the main of elderly victims, often living alone. The difficulties which faced such victims after their injury may be assumed to be of a somewhat different nature from those which would be expected in a sample of victims normally responsible for providing the household income or looking after young children. This is reflected in the lack of information relating to income and employment difficulties suffered by victims. Since many were receiving state retirement pensions, their finances were not affected by an inability to carry on as normal. Often our elderly victims were, before the accident, already receiving some kind of supportive assistance from both formal and informal sources and thus the effects of their accidents were to some extent cushioned by this existing support.

Where respondents were working at the time of the accident, time off work frequently resulted in loss of income, although this loss of income did not necessarily cause major disruptions in the household.

However, when a housewife with a family at home suffered from lengthy functional difficulties, her normal tasks had to be taken over by others, involving considerable informal reorganisation. We see that this is generally done by family, friends and neighbours rather than by official agencies. On the whole it is the elderly who make use of formal supporting services.

The legal questions asked of our victims have demonstrated clearly the relatively slight use made of the legal system by home accident victims, and indeed the infrequency with which victims even consider turning to the law to gain compensation for injuries suffered in domestic accidents.

The Bristol study has provided useful experience for further development of research concerning the consequences of injury from accidents in the home, and raised questions which the Centre for Socio-Legal Studies will explore in the course of its national survey of misfortune.

Notes

1. For children, we included going to school, playing and normal self-care.
2. We would like to acknowledge the cooperation and assistance given to us by the Medical Research Division in Bristol of the Health Education Council, in particular Dr J. W. Dale.
3. This finding may have important implications for the national surveillance system (see above, Chapter 4a-d), since such victims would never appear in any statistics collected from hospitals.

References

Alphey, R. S. and Leach, S. J. (1974) *Accidental Death in the Home.* Building Research Establishment Current Paper, CP 98/74. Garston: BRE Building Research Station.

Burman, S. B., Genn, H. G. and Lyons, J. (1977) Pilot study of the use of legal services by victims of accidents in the home. *Modern Law Review,* **40** (forthcoming).

Genn, H. G. and Burman, S. B. (1976) Report of a Pilot Study of Home Accident Victims. Oxford: Centre for Socio-Legal Studies. Mimeo.

Maclean, M. and Genn, H. G. (1975) Informal service relationships following accidents in the home. Paper presented to Medical Sociology Subsection of British Sociological Association Conference, York. Mimeo.

Phillips, J. and Hawkins, K. (1976) Some economic aspects of the settlement process: a study of personal injury claims. *Modern Law Review,* 39, No. 4, 497-515.

Thomson, J. and Hesketh, L. J. (1975) Accident Surveillance System for Home Accidents. Home Office and Department of Prices and Consumer Protection paper. London: DPCP. Mimeo.

APPENDIX: CONFERENCE ON SOCIAL, ECONOMIC AND LEGAL ASPECTS OF ACCIDENTS IN THE HOME

Wolfson College, Oxford: 29-30 June 1976

List of Conference Participants

Professor E. Maurice BACKETT, Department of Community Health, University of Nottingham

Dr Alan BEATTIE, Department of Community Health, University of Nottingham

Dr John BREAUX, Department of Psychology, University of Surrey

Dr Sandra BURMAN, Centre for Socio-Legal Studies, University of Oxford

Mr Michael CALNAN, National Children's Bureau

Dr David CANTER, Department of Psychology, University of Surrey

Mr A. J. CLARK, Department of the Environment Building Research Station, Garston

Mr Peter CORFIELD, Centre for Socio-Legal Studies, University of Oxford

Dr John W. DALE, St Thomas' Department of Community Medicine, Sussex

Dr C. P. de FONSEKA, Royal United Hospital, Bath

Mr Michael DUNNE, Research Institute of Consumer Affairs

Ms Hazel GENN, Centre for Socio-Legal Studies, University of Oxford

Mr Donald HARRIS, Centre for Socio-Legal Studies, University of Oxford

Ms Louise HESKETH, Home Office Scientific Advisory Branch

Dr R. H. JACKSON, Department of Child Health, University of Newcastle upon Tyne

Ms Judith LITTLEWOOD, Department of the Environment Social Research Division

Dr Sally LLOYD-BOSTOCK, Centre for Socio-Legal Studies, University of Oxford

Dr Bronwen LODER, Medical Research Council

Ms Mavis MACLEAN, Centre for Socio-Legal Studies, University of Oxford

Mr Bob PAGE, Department of Prices and Consumer Protection Safety Research Section

Ms Jenny PHILLIPS, Centre for Socio-Legal Studies, University of

Oxford

Dr John ROBERTS, South Glamorgan Health Authority

Mr St John SANDRINGHAM, Consumers' Association

Mr Ned SCOTT, British Market Research Bureau

Mr Jonathan SIME, Department of Psychology, University of Surrey

Dr David STURROCK, Medical Research Council

Ms Jane THOMAS, Health Education Council

Ms Susan TRYNER, Department of Prices and Consumer Protection
Safety Research Section

Ms Caroline WARNE, Department of Prices and Consumer Protection
Safety Research Section

Dr G. M. B. WEBBER, Department of the Environment Building
Research Station, Garston

Ms Heather WHICHER, Lincoln's Inn, London

Ms Claire WHITTINGTON, Institute for Consumer Ergonomics,
Loughborough

Mr J. R. WILSON, Institute for Consumer Ergonomics, Loughborough

INDEX

137